C0-GHA-638

Nutrition in the Young and the Elderly

Nutrition in the Young and the Elderly:

A Symposium Held at the School of Medicine University of Minnesota, Duluth June 28–30, 1982

Edited by

Edwin W. Haller, Ph.D.
Department of Physiology
University of Minnesota, Duluth

Gerald E. Cotton, M.D.
Department of Clinical Sciences
University of Minnesota, Duluth

THE COLLAMORE PRESS
D.C. Heath and Company
Lexington, Massachusetts
Toronto

ST. PHILIP'S COLLEGE LIBRARY

Every effort has been made to ensure that drug dosage schedules and indications are correct at the time of publication. Since ongoing medical research can change standards of usage, and also because of human and typographical error, it is recommended that readers check the *PDR* or package insert before prescription or administration of the drugs mentioned in this book.

RC
620.5
.N863
1983

Copyright © 1983 by D.C. Heath Company

All rights reserved. No part of this publication may be reproduced or transmitted in any form or by any means, electronic or mechanical, including photocopy, recording, or any information storage or retrieval system, without permission in writing from the publisher.

Published simultaneously in Canada

Printed in the United States of America

International Standard Book Number: 0-669-06341-X

Library of Congress Catalog Card Number: 82-73329

Library of Congress Cataloging in Publication Data
Main entry under title:

Nutrition in the young and the elderly.

Includes bibliographies and index.
1. Nutrition disorders—Congresses. 2. Aged—Nutrition—Congresses. 3. Youth—Nutrition—Congresses. I. Haller, Edwin W. II. Cotton, Gerald E. [DNLM: 1. Nutrition—In old age—Congresses. 2. Child nutrition—Congresses.
QU 145 N97531 1982]
RC620.5.N863 1983 616.3'9 82-73329
ISBN 0-669-06341-X

Contents

081894

Preface

The fourth annual symposium on "Medical Research: Pathway to Better Health" was held in Duluth on June 28–30, 1982. This year's topic, "Nutrition in the Young and the Elderly," was particularly timely for several reasons. Increased awareness by the health professions of the need for better nutrition education, greater recognition of the important relationships between nutrition, healing, and health, the abundance of inaccurate nutrition information in the public sector, and acceptance of the leading role of health professionals in forming public opinion and social policy have all combined to focus on the nutritional needs of the fragile portions of our society: the young and elderly.

The symposium and its proceedings were organized into five topical sections that dealt with areas of specific interest concerning nutritional needs of the young and elderly populations. Each section was concluded by a panel discussion in which both the speakers of the section and the audience participated. This provided an opportunity to all participants of the symposium to offer many valuable additional points. Therefore, a narrative synopsis of each of these discussions is included at the end of each section. A summation of the major conclusions that resulted from the symposium is presented at the end of the proceedings.

The symposium was conceived as a means to enliven the discussion between researcher and provider of health care, between academician and practitioner. We hope this purpose was achieved. And we hope that by the publication of these proceedings the spirit of awareness will transcend the immediacy of the symposium to translate the continuing quest for better health care into concrete action.

The organization of a symposium requires much support and commitment of time by many. We want to take this opportunity to express our thanks. The School of Medicine at the University of Minnesota, Duluth, graciously hosted the symposium and gave generous support from its resources. Major contributions were received from the Duluth Clinic Education and Research Foundation and the Miller-Dwan Medical Center Foundation of Duluth. Additional grants were provided by the St. Luke's Hospital Foundation of Duluth and by the following industries: Ross Laboratories, Mead-Johnson Pharmaceuticals, Norwich-Eaton Company, USV Laboratories, the Upjohn Company, and Deluxe Check Printers. Most important, however, the enthusiastic support of many unnamed individuals made the symposium possible. We would like to thank especially Paul C. Royce, Dean of the School of Medicine; the organizing committee for the symposium; and the faculty and staff of the School of Medicine. Lynn Devlin, Janet DeRoche, Donna Kotter, and Diana Buck handled the seemingly unending paperwork and typing cheerfully and with ease, and Mark Summers lent his professional skill to assure a flawless performance of the audiovisual equipment. Our thanks go to all who helped.

E.W.H.
G.E.C.

Contributing Authors

Roslyn B. Alfin-Slater, Ph.D.
Professor of Nutrition
School of Public Health
University of California
Los Angeles

George L. Blackburn, M.D., Ph.D.
Director, Nutrition Support Service
Director, Nutrition Metabolism Laboratory
New England Deaconess Hospital
Boston, Massachusetts

Nathaniel G. Clark, M.S., R.D.
Clinical Dietitian in Hyperalimentation
Research Associate, Nutrition and Metabolism
Nutrition Support Service
Cancer Research Institute
New England Deaconess Hospital
Boston, Massachusetts

Mary Darling, M.P.H., R.D.
Assistant Professor and Extension Nutritionist
Department of Food Science and Nutrition
Agriculture Extension Service
University of Minnesota
St. Paul

Hector F. DeLuca, Ph.D.
Professor and Chairman
Department of Biochemistry
University of Wisconsin
Madison

Stephen P. Fortmann, M.D.
Assistant Professor of Medicine
Stanford Heart Disease Prevention Program
Stanford University
Stanford, California

Clifford F. Gastineau, M.D., Ph.D.
Professor of Medicine
The Mayo Clinic
Rochester, Minnesota

Saxon Graham, Ph.D.
Professor and Chairman
Department of Social and Preventive Medicine
State University of New York
Buffalo

Patrick V.J. Hegarty, Ph.D.
Professor of Nutrition
Department of Food Science and Nutrition
University of Minnesota
St. Paul

Victor Herbert, M.D., J.D.
Professor of Medicine
State University of New York, Downstate Medical Center
Brooklyn
Chief, Hematology and Nutrition Laboratory
Veterans Administration Medical Center
Bronx

Barbara K. Herzog, Ph.D.
Division of Legislation, Research and Developmental Services
American Association of Retired Persons
Washington, DC

Robert E. Hodges, M.D.
Head, Clinical Nutrition Division
Department of Internal Medicine
University of Nebraska Medical Center
Omaha

William F. Hueg, Jr., Ph.D.
Professor and Dean
Institute of Agriculture, Forestry and Home Economics
University of Minnesota
St. Paul

Paul A. Kerschner, Ph.D.
Associate Director
Division of Legislation, Research and Developmental Services
American Association of Retired Persons
Washington, DC

Richard S. Rivlin, M.D.
Professor of Medicine and Chief, Nutrition Service
Memorial Sloan-Kettering Cancer Center
and New York Hospital–Cornell Medical Center
New York

Meinhard Robinow, M.D.
Director of Dysmorphology
The Children's Medical Center
Dayton, Ohio

Daphne A. Roe, M.D.
Professor of Nutrition
Cornell University
Ithaca, New York

Patricia B. Swan, Ph.D.
Professor of Nutrition
Department of Food Science and Nutrition
University of Minnesota
St. Paul

Eleanor A. Young, Ph.D., R.D.
Associate Professor
Division of Gastroenterology and Nutrition
Department of Medicine
University of Texas Health Science Center
San Antonio

I Definition of the Problem

1 Nutrition and Health: Their Interrelationships in the Young and the Old

Robert E. Hodges, M.D.

Many years ago a well-known physician, nutritionist, and investigator named Paul Gyorgy used to comment on the "late effects of early nutrition." He studied children not only in his hometown of Philadelphia but also in many parts of the world, especially Indonesia. He was convinced that childhood malnutrition resulted in latent defects that eventually would become apparent if the individual lived long enough.

In this introductory chapter I will discuss the historical events that led step by step to our modern concepts of nutrition and health and to the present-day evidence that certain forms of malnutrition, even though mild and completely asymptomatic, may result in tragic disease decades later.

Basis for Modern Concepts of Nutrition and Disease

A predictable characteristic of government is that they are very apt to "grease the wheel that squeaks the loudest." This may explain the fact that three successive wars resulted in the creation, by the United States government, of three agencies designed to collect scientific information and provide the best advice available regarding nutrition and health, but that in peacetime there was little progress. In the early days of the Civil War, the National Academy of Sciences was founded. Among their many tasks was the assignment to estimate the food requirements of the armed forces of the North. At that time foods were known to contain protein, carbohydrates, and fats, but vitamins had not yet been discovered.

With the outbreak of World War I, the government saw fit to found the National Research Council, which was charged with the responsibility of determining how much food would be needed and how much was available at that time. The Allies, particularly Britain and France, were desperately short of food supplies and required aid from the United States. By this time the first of the vitamins had been discovered. A substance called "fat-soluble A" was found, and soon after "water-soluble B" was identified. During the war years and shortly thereafter, several additional vitamins were identified and their nutritional roles were at least partially elucidated.

With the commencement of hostilities in Europe in the late 1930s, the United States once again realized that we were soon to be called upon to provide food and nutritional counseling to the Allied forces and before long to our own forces. By this time nutrition had become much more of a science, and the Food and Nutrition Board was created by the government. However, instead of being concerned chiefly with gross amounts of food or with food supplies that contained adequate amounts of the vitamins and essential minerals, the board was now concerned with concentrated food supplies that could be easily carried, would not require cooking facilities, and would require no refrigeration for long periods of time. Perhaps no other rations were detested so wholeheartedly by the armed forces as these rations. An interesting fact is that each packet of K-rations also contained cigarettes, along with instant coffee, a sweetened dehydrated lemonade or a chocolate-flavored disk that could be made into something resembling hot chocolate, a few crackers or biscuits, and a sealed metal container of processed meat or cheese as a protein food. The fact that the troops often discarded these metal containers unopened attests to their unpalatability. No doubt many men in our Armed Forces were inadequately fed for varying periods of time when they were issued these rations. In addition, the ubiquitous cigarettes were provided free, and there were few who did not smoke them. Now, 40 years later, we see vast numbers of men in our Veterans Administration Hospitals who have chronic obstructive lung disease, lung cancer, and coronary heart disease, in part as a result of smoking. But we shall see later that these illnesses, along with high blood pressure and stroke, may have been worsened by diet.

International surveys of children in developing countries tell us that malnutrition greatly enhances susceptibility to infection and retards growth. In our own country, available statistics on food consumption and causes of death disclose interesting correlations. In 1900 influenza and pneumonia headed the list of causes of death, with 203 deaths per 100,000. By 1955 this had fallen to 27 and by 1979, to 20. No doubt the discovery of antibiotics and the sophisticated techniques available in modern hospitals accounted for much of this improvement. Similarly, tuberculosis was the second most common cause of death in 1900, with 202 cases per 100,000, whereas in 1955 it had fallen to 9 and in 1979, to 1. Diarrhea and enteritis came next, with 133 cases in 1900 and 5 cases in 1955. This category was not listed in 1979. Most deaths from diarrhea result from lack of sanitation and lack of available antibiotics. Diseases of the heart, not including coronary artery disease, accounted for 132 deaths per 100,000 in 1900, 108 in 1955, and only 81 in 1979. But coronary artery disease, which was not even listed in 1900 or 1955, accounted for 250 deaths per 100,000 in 1979. Stroke, which accounted for 72 deaths per 100,000 in 1900, rose to 106 in 1955 and declined to 77 in 1979. Cancer, which may not have been accurately diagnosed in earlier days, was listed as causing 63 deaths per 100,000 in 1900 and more than double that amount, 146, in 1955 [1]. By 1979 this had risen to 184.

If we examine age-adjusted cancer death rates for men and women in the United States, we find that cancer, in general, continues to be a common disease, second only to coronary heart disease as a cause of death. But there are three noteworthy changes. The first of these is a gratifying fall in deaths from cancer of the uterus, which almost certainly resulted from the success of the Papanicolaou smear. The second is the dramatic and tragic rise in deaths from lung cancer in men, and more recently, a similar trend in women. We know that cigarette smoking causes lung cancer, but recent evidence implicates nutritional factors as well [2,3]. The third impressive change in cancer statistics is the decisive decrease in death rate from stomach cancer in both men and women between 1930 and 1980 [4]. This change also may be related to the food we eat [5]: it may be explained by reduced consumption of nitrates and smoked foods.

Thus, for at least the past two decades, there have been three major killers in the United States: coronary artery disease, cancer, and stroke. As we shall see, there is reason to believe that diet may be a contributing factor in all three.

Influence of Nutrition on Health in Later Life

Nutrition in Pregnancy and Effect on the Fetus

Certain events occurring early in pregnancy may be reflected in the health of individuals 20 or more years later. In some instances, the defects may persist throughout life. This is true of the fetal alcohol syndrome, which is characterized by typical abnormalities of the facial structures, mental deficiencies, and certain abnormalities of the musculoskeletal system [6]. This tragic syndrome may result from lack of proper food because the mother cannot afford both alcoholic beverages and food, from the effects of ethanol on certain vitamins such as folic acid, or from toxicity of alcohol itself. In pregnant animals, starvation ketosis causes an increase in embryonic deaths and a variety of congenital deformities. Specific nutrient deficiency syndromes that can be teratogenic in animals include lack of folic acid, vitamin A, riboflavin, or pantothenic acid. In addition, deficiency of zinc is highly teratogenic [7].

A classic study of starvation during pregnancy [8] led to some surprising information about adipocytes and body habitus. During the closing months of World War II the Allies attempted to shorten the war by dropping paratroopers into parts of Holland, where they were expected to capture a bridge across the Rhine and disrupt the Nazi retreat to Berlin [9,10]. Many factors combined to make this attempt a disaster. Subsequently the Germans, in order to punish the Dutch population for their collaboration with the British and Americans, sharply reduced the amount of food available to each citizen of certain localities in Holland. Of course, a certain number of pregnancies occurred during this time, and approximately 30 years after the war a group of investigators from the United States chose to study the survivors of this period of starvation. Because the Dutch have always been meticulous record keepers, it was possible to locate almost everyone who had been born during or subsequent to the Nazi punishment of these villagers. Although the investigators did not find evidence that semistarvation in utero or in the early neonatal period produced objective evidence of mental impairment, they did find, much to their surprise, that the offspring of pregnant women who were deprived of adequate food early in the course of pregnancy, when the neurologic system was being formed, became obese in adult life. By contrast, the offspring of women who were semistarved during the last months of pregnancy—and particularly if the newborn babies received inadequate nourishment—became unusually lean adults. The investigators speculated that when the semistarvation occurred early in pregnancy, there was imperfect formation of the child's hypothalamic centers that control appetite. Conversely, when starvation occurred late in pregnancy or early in extrauterine life, the numbers of fat cells produced by the fetus or newborn child were presumably less than average. Thus an event occurring in utero may well have a significant impact on the health of an individual when he or she reaches adult age.

Another event that can occur in pregnancy may have an important impact on the health of the offspring: megadoses of vitamin A [11], vitamin D [12], or vitamin C can produce malformation of the offspring or may even disrupt the pregnancy. Excessive doses of vitamin A given to pregnant experimental animals may cause malformation of facial structures, particularly the eyes. An overdose of vitamin D given to a pregnant animal can cause cardiac malformations. Even vitamin C can be toxic when given in very large amounts. Studies in both experimental animals and humans have shown that large doses of ascorbic acid can disrupt pregnancy or can result in malformation [13].

Nutrition in Infancy and Childhood

Children form their patterns of eating in their own homes. If a child is exposed to a family that gathers together at the breakfast table every day, the chances are reasonably good that he will grow up to enjoy breakfast and the nutrients it provides. On the other hand, in a family where the situation is "everyone for himself," many people find it easier to skip breakfast than to pour a glass of orange juice and eat a bowl of cereal with milk. Since breakfast is the only meal that is likely to include substantial amounts of both vitamin C and vitamin A, the result may be marginal or deficient levels of intake of these two vitamins throughout a lifetime. Because so many people live at a distance from their place of employment, lunch in the United States has become largely a meal eaten away from home. This situation, of course, favors the proliferation of fast-food establishments and the high-caloric items they sell. Furthermore, many fast-food stores do not offer a salad, which could measurably improve the quality of nutrition, and many fast foods are quite salty. Dinner, the only meal of the day at which the family is likely to congregate, is an opportunity to make up for some of the deficits during the day and may make a significant difference in the nutritional health of an individual.

An astonishing report from Holland suggests strongly that early nutrition has a great impact on later health. Dijkstra [3] studied 330 cases of bronchial cancer occurring between January 1, 1950, and January 1, 1960. Much to his surprise, he discovered that there was a seasonal effect on incidence, which he explained by the absence of vitamin A, or rather of carotene, in the diet of children born during the winter months as compared with children born during the summer months. He postulated that the epithelium of the respiratory tract may be incompletely formed at birth, and so ample amounts of vitamin A might be needed to permit normal maturation of this epithelium [3]. In any event, his statistical comparisons are very convincing and fit in nicely with the observations of Shekelle and colleagues [2], who studied a large number of adults in Chicago. These researchers were studying primarily diet and coronary heart disease, but they were also interested in any aspects of health that were influenced by diet. As expected, they found that cigarette smokers had a much higher incidence of lung cancer than did nonsmokers, but an unexpected finding was the very pronounced effect of dietary carotene on lung cancer: those individuals who consumed the most carotene had the lowest prevalence of lung cancer, and vice versa. The consumption of carotene was estimated by questionnaires that determined the amounts of salads, soups, and fruits consumed by the subjects in this study.

Relationship of Diet and Disease in the Adult

The National Research Council recently released a report prepared by an expert committee which compared the effects of diet and nutrition on cancer [14]. Release of their recommendations has resulted in sharp polarization of scientists and lay people alike. On the one hand, people are saying that our food supply is the best in the world and so is the health of our population—

why should we attempt to change our diet now? On the other hand, the incidence of several different types of cancer has been correlated with certain characteristics of our diet, and presumably a change of diet could reduce the prevalence of these cancers.

If we look at the dietary changes that have occurred in the United States since 1900, we find that civilian consumption of major food commodities per person showed a moderate rise between 1910 and 1955 [15], with a continuing rise into 1970 and 1980 [16]. Dairy products, including butter, rose substantially between 1910 and 1955, but the consumption of butter fell sharply by 1980, whereas consumption of cheese doubled between 1960 and 1980. At the same time fruits and vegetables, which rose markedly from 1910 to 1945, began to decline by 1950 and continued their downward trend into the 1970s. Fresh vegetables have also been less popular in recent decades, with frozen potatoes edging out fresh potatoes by a substantial margin. Similarly, consumption of cereal products and grains declined between 1910 and 1960 but leveled off in recent years. Consumption of sugar rose rapidly after the turn of the century but has been essentially unchanged in recent decades, except for a transient fall during the war years. At the same time, consumption of fats, as a percentage of total calories consumed, rose from about 30 percent to 40 or even 42 percent of our diet. Another change that has occurred is a reduction in the amount of smoked and salted meats that we consume and a reduction in the amount of nitrates added to hams, bacon, and other meats [4].

Epidemiologically, some of our commoner forms of cancer have been correlated with dietary fat, whereas coronary heart disease has been correlated with high concentrations of cholesterol in the plasma [17]. Furthermore, dietary sodium has, in most studies, been correlated with a rise in blood pressure. Blood pressure in turn is closely related to the risk of stroke.

Current Health Status of Americans

Despite all the factors mentioned here, the health of most people in the United States must be considered to be very good indeed. Reproduction occurs at a steady rate and with very few complications. Average life expectancy at birth is 69.9 years for boys and 77.8 years for girls. The rate of growth of American children is very high compared with children of the developing countries, where food supplies are limited. Life expectancy of men and women at age 50 is approximately 30 years, but the spectrum of causes of death remains the same, with coronary heart disease heading the list, followed by cancer and then stroke.

After examining the report issued by the National Research Council, one might pose the following six questions:

1. Does diet affect serum lipids?
2. Do serum lipids affect the incidence of coronary heart disease and stroke?
3. Do sodium and potassium in the diet affect blood pressure?
4. Does elevated blood pressure affect the death rate from stroke?
5. Do dietary components affect the incidence of cancer?
6. Would dietary changes be likely to decrease cancer deaths?

Final answers to these questions will be slow in coming. A good analogy is the scientific turmoil that existed 20 years ago when epidemiologists and others suggested that lung cancer could result from smoking cigarettes. This has been determined to be true, but it took many years to answer this question.

Summary

The diet consumed by the average person in the United States has been changing constantly, at least since 1900. During this time, causes of death also have changed remarkably. Some of these changes are unlikely to be related to diet. Some late effects of early nutrition can carry through a lifetime. Furthermore, certain childhood habits may persist throughout life, including skipping breakfast, excessive use of salt, fondness for sweets, dislike of salads and fresh fruits and vegetables, and preference for fatty foods such as butter, gravy, ice cream, cheese, and frankfurters. The answers to the questions raised in this summary are currently uncertain, and will no doubt remain so for many years. Nonetheless, we must explore many possibilities if we are to achieve improvement in our national health.

References

1. Cancer statistics, 1982. *Ca—A Cancer Journal for Clinicians* 32:15–31, 1982.

2. Shekelle, R.B., Lepper, M., Shugney, L., et al. Dietary vitamin A and risk of cancer in the Western Electric study. *Lancet* 2:1185–1189, 1981.

3. Dijkstra, B.K.S. Origin of carcinoma of the bronchus. *J. Natl. Cancer Inst.* 11:511–519, 1963.

4. MacGregor, I.L. Carcinoma of the colon and stomach. *J.A.M.A.* 227: 911–915, 1974.

5. Green, L.C., Tannenbaum, S.R. Nitrate and nitrite in food. *Nutrition and the M.D.* 8(5):1–3, 1982.

6. Hanson, J.W., Smith, D.W., Jones, K.S. Fetal alcohol syndrome. *J.A.M.A.* 235:1458–1460, 1976.

7. Giroud, A. *The Nutrition of the Embryo*. Springfield, Ill.: Charles C Thomas, 1970.

8. Roeder, L.M., Chow, B.F. Maternal undernutrition and its long-term effects on the offspring. *Am. J. Clin. Nutr.* 25:812–821, 1972.

9. Ravelli, G.P., Stein, Z.A., Susser, M.W. Obesity in young men after famine exposure in utero and early infancy. *N. Engl. J. Med.* 295:349–353, 1976.

10. Stein, Z., Susser, M., Saenger, G., Marolla, F. *Famine and Human Development: The Dutch Hunger-Winter of 1944–1945*. New York: Oxford University Press, 1975.

11. Kalter, H., Warkang, J. Experimental production of congenital malformations in strains of inbred mice by maternal treatment with hypervitaminosis A. *Am. J. Pathol.* 38:1–21, 1961.

12. Friedman, W.F., Roberts, W.C. Vitamin D and the supravalvular aortic stenosis syndrome. *Circulation* 34:77–86, 1966.

13. Samborskaya, E.P., Ferdman, T.D. Mechanism of termination of pregnancy by ascorbic acid. *Bulleten Eksperimental Noi Biologii i Medicin* 62:96–98, 1966.

14. *Diet, Nutrition and Cancer.* Committee on Diet, Nutrition and Cancer, Assembly of Life Sciences, and National Research Council. Washington, D.C.: National Academy Press, 1982

15. Antar, M.A., Ohlson, M.A., Hodges, E. Changes in retail market food supplies in the United States in the last seventy years in relation to the incidence of coronary heart disease, with special reference to dietary carbohydrates and essential fatty acids. *Am. J. Clin. Nutr.* 14:169–178, 1964.

16. Economics Research Service. Civilian consumption of major food commodities per person, 1960, 1980. U.S. Department of Agriculture. Quoted in *The World Almanac and Book of Facts, 1982*. New York: Newspaper Enterprise Association, 1982.

17. Kannel, W.B. Meaning of the downward trend in cardiovascular mortality. *J.A.M.A.* 247:877–880, 1982.

2 Nutritional Assessment of the Elderly Institutionalized Patient

Nathaniel G. Clark, M.S.
George L. Blackburn, M.D., Ph.D.

The correct and accurate nutritional assessment of the institutionalized elderly patient depends on an understanding of three factors: the techniques of nutritional assessment presently in use clinically, the effects of aging on nutritional status, and the effects of institutionalization (and inactivity) on nutritional status. This patient population has unique needs and therefore requires quite specialized assessment tools and standards.

The U.S. Census Bureau's 1977 projection of what the nation's population aged 65 and over would be by the year 2000 was 31.8 million (Table 2-1). Declining birth rates coupled with modest increases in longevity have brought about a new interest in caring for the elderly, who may constitute 12–15 percent of the U.S. population by the year 2000. Perhaps 50 percent of these will be 75 or older.

Characteristically, the elderly undergo declining health and increased use of health care services. They are bedridden twice as many days as those 45–64 years old, spend three times as many days in acute care centers, and have a length of stay almost twice that of younger persons (Table 2-2). During 1977 about 11 percent of the population was 65 or older but accounted for 29 per-

Table 2–1
U.S. Population: 1960–2020

Year	*Population (millions)*	*Percentage Under 15*	*Percentage 65 or Older*	*Percentage 75 or Older*
1960	181	31.0	9.2	3.1
1980	222	22.5	11.2	4.2
2000 (est.)	260	21.9	12.2	5.5
2020 (est.)	290	20.7	15.5	5.9

Source: United States Census and Projections.
(est.) = estimated.

This research was supported in part by a grant from the Center for Nutritional Research Charitable Trust.

Table 2–2
Annual Acute Hospitalization Utilization, By Age

Age Group	*Hospitalization Rate (per 1,000)*	*Days of Acute Care (per person)*	*Average Length of Stay (days)*
All ages	163	1.3	7.7
55-64 years	215	2.1	9.7
65 and over	359	4.2	11.6
64-74 years	300	3.3	11.1
Over 75 years	463	4.6	12.2

Source: Vital and Health Statistics, series 13, no. 31, 1977.

Table 2–3
Expenditures For Personal Health Care (Fiscal Year 1977)

Expenditures	*Under Age 65*	*Age 65 and Older*
Total, per capita	$514	$1,745
Source		
Direct payment	32%	27%
Private health insurance	36%	6%
Government	29%	67%
Philanthropy and industry	3%	1%

Source: From a compilation by the Health Care Financing Administration, *Health in the United States*, 1979.

cent of the total health care dollars spent in the United States. Almost 66 percent of those health care dollars came from the public sector (Table 2-3).

As the elderly segment of our population continues to increase, so will the institutionalized segment. At this time approximately 3 percent of elderly persons 65–74 years old are in institutions. Estimates of the number of nursing home residents per 1,000 population project an increase from 6.0 in 1980 to 12.2 in 2040 (a 100 percent increase).

Nutritional assessment is best thought of as consisting of the choice of appropriate tests and appropriate standards for their interpretation. What is becoming very clear as more and more elderly patient populations are assessed is that while many of the assessment techniques that have been used for some time in younger patients have direct application to elderly patients as well, the choice of appropriate standards is very difficult. No standards presently exist for this population group, and for this reason some possible new standards will be discussed here.

In this chapter we will discuss the techniques of nutritional assessment currently in use; the aging process and its effect on body composition, metabolism and nutritional/metabolic parameters; some results of our laboratory research on the nutritional assessment of chronically ill, hospitalized patients both as a group and also when compared to free-living, healthy elderly persons; and finally, the prognostic power of nutritional assessment in determining patient health outcome.

Nutritional Assessment Techniques

The nutritional and metabolic assessment of the hospitalized patient has been presented in detail [1]. Briefly, the patient is assessed by the use of anthropometric, laboratory, and immunologic tests.

Anthropometrics

Height and *weight*, while still too difficult to obtain on all hospitalized patients, provide useful information about the patient's energy status. The *percentage of ideal weight for height* is calculated using "ideal" weight/height tables. In addition to simply noting the patient's weight (and percentage of ideal), one needs to determine the *weight history*, documenting any recent losses (or gains) in weight that were not planned. Both the amount of weight lost and the time involved are critical, as seen in Table 2-4.

One next determines the *triceps skinfold* and the *arm muscle circumference*, which document the status of the patient's body fat and somatic (muscle) protein status, respectively. Published standards for hospitalized patients in general exist for the interpretation of these tests [1].

Laboratory Tests

The laboratory assessment is based on the levels of albumin and transferrin in the blood and creatinine and urea nitrogen in a 24-hour urine specimen.

Table 2-4
Evaluation of Weight Change[a]

Time	*Significant Weight Loss (%)*	*Severe Weight Loss (%)*
1 week	1-2	>2
1 month	5	>5
3 months	7.5	>7.5
6 months	10	>10

Source: Compiled from Blackburn et al. [1].
[a]Values charted are for percentage of weight change:

$$\text{Percentage of Weight Change} = \frac{(\text{Usual weight} - \text{Actual weight})}{(\text{Usual weight})} \times 100.$$

Albumin (half-life, 20 days) and transferrin (half-life, 8 days) levels allow one to assess the visceral protein status of the patient on a long-term and short-term basis, respectively. The urinary urea nitrogen level gives information both on the patient's level of catabolic stress [2] and on the amount of protein the patient is metabolizing, whether it is endogenous or exogenous.

Urinary creatinine has been shown to be an excellent index of total body muscle mass as well as lean body mass [3]. One can calculate the patient's *creatinine height index* by comparing the patient's 24-hour excretion of creatinine to the published theoretical "ideal" excretion for a person of the same height [4]. With the information gathered from the anthropometric and laboratory tests cited above, one can quite objectively assess the nutritional status of the hospitalized patient. What remains to be done is to examine the *effects* of the nutritional status by assessing the immune system.

Immunologic Tests

Since lymphocytes are an important part of the body's immune system, the calculation of the *total lymphocyte count* using the white blood cell count and the differential is very important. We can specifically measure the delayed hypersensitivity immune response by the use of *recall skin antigen tests.* Here the patient is challenged with common antigens (*Candida*, mumps) placed intradermally to which the patient either reacts (>5 mm induration or redness) or not.

Changes in Body Composition

The aging process results in characteristic changes in body composition and metabolism, which have been well reviewed by Munro [5]. With the aging process comes a decrease in lean body mass, the metabolically active and vital portion of the body. Using ^{40}K analysis, Forbes has documented a decrease of 6.3 percent per decade [6]. In terms of specific tissues, the following decreases in tissue weight have been noted: muscle, 40 percent; kidney, 9 percent; liver, 18 percent; and lung, 11 percent [7]. These changes obviously have profound implications on nutrient requirements, metabolism, and excretion. With this decrease in lean body mass comes approximately a 30 percent increase in total body fat. Given these changes, a patient's weight must be considered carefully. Although he or she may weigh the same at 75 as at 35 years, the composition of that weight (and therefore nutrient requirements) will be very different.

In addition, a decrease in bone mass in the elderly has been documented [8]. Men appear to have a decrease of approximately 12 percent and women,

25 percent in total bone mass. This reduction in bone mass is demonstrated in the proclivity of the elderly population toward spontaneous fractures. The etiology of the decreased bone mass is not clear, and the role that nutrition plays in its occurrence or could play in its treatment is a matter of much debate. What can be said is that hormone shifts, progressive inactivity, and nutrition are all important factors.

Accompanying these changes in body composition are changes in metabolism, which are closely linked to the body composition changes noted above. Basal energy expenditure, the amount of energy needed to maintain the body in its basal state without activity or stress, decreases 20 percent per unit of surface area between 30 and 90 years of age [9]. It is important to note, however, that there is no change in basal energy expenditure per unit of active tissue. What is seen is a primary decrease in lean body mass leading to a secondary decrease in basal energy expenditure.

Changes in Protein Metabolism

Protein metabolism also is affected by aging. Total synthesis and breakdown are seen to decrease [10], again due to a decreased lean body (protein) mass. Muscle protein metabolism shifts as a result of shrinking muscle mass, as already noted. While a decrease in breakdown of muscle protein (using the excretion of 3-methylhistidine, a nonreutilized amino acid, as an index) is seen per kilogram of body weight, no decrease is seen per unit of creatinine (an index of muscle mass) [11]. Again what is demonstrated is that a decreasing protein mass is leading to a decrease in turnover; what is decreasing is not the *rate* but the total *amount* of turnover.

Visceral protein metabolism (seen by examining albumin metabolism) also undergoes changes [12]. It appears that the elderly have a lower synthetic rate that is not as responsive to changes in protein intake as in younger persons. Levels of serum albumin have been noted to be decreased in some studies of the elderly, and this may be a partial cause. Alternatively, others have noted that hypoalbuminemic patients have an increased catabolic rate [13].

Changes in Nutritional Assessment Parameters

Having considered the currently utilized nutritional assessment techniques and the effects of aging on nutrition and metabolism, we now turn to the effects of aging on the commonly measured nutritional assessment parameters and suggest standards that take these changes into account (see Table 2-5).

Table 2–5
Standards For Nutritional Assessment of the Elderly

	Anthropometrics[a]		
	Males		*Females*
Arm muscle circumference (AMC)[b]	26.8		22.5
Triceps skinfold (TSF) (mm)[b]	11.0		24.0
	Laboratory Tests (% of Deficit)		
Blood tests	*Mild*	*Moderate*	*Severe*
Albumin (g/dl)[c]	3.5–3.2	3.2–2.8	<2.8
Transferrin (mg/dl)[c]	200–180	180–160	<160
Total lymphocyte count (no/mm^3)[c]	1800–1500	1500–900	<900
Urine tests			
Urinary creatinine (g/24 hr)	According to height (see reference [4])		

[a] For weight/height percentiles, see Figure 2–1. For evaluation of weight loss, see Table 2–4.

[b] Data from Frisancho [18].

[c] Data from Blackburn [26].

Anthropometrics

Height. Stature is felt to decrease with aging, most likely as a result of a gradual narrowing of the spinal disk structures and shortened vertebral heights [14]. Long-bone length appears to be more stable and may provide a new and improved tool for future studies [15].

Weight. The average weight for a given height has been documented to increase with aging. Analysis of the 1971–1974 Health and Nutrition Examination Survey (HANES) data reveals a steady increase with aging in the mean weight for a given height until the fifth and sixth decades [16] and then a decline [17]. Within the elderly age range especially, Master et al. [17] have documented a steady decrease in weight for height from 64 years of age to 94 years of age. If one keeps in mind the changes in body composition that occur with aging (decreased lean body mass, increased total body fat), the concept of "ideal weight for height" becomes quite complex. Clearly, what one wants to maintain or replenish is lean body mass, not body fat, so the measurement of weight must be accompanied by tests of lean body status. Designing a useful standard of weight for height in the elderly institutionalized patient is, however, very important.

From the HANES, it is now possible to find the fifth through ninety-fifth percentile values for the weight of an elderly person at any given height. In Figure 2-1, the fifth and fiftieth percentiles are shown. The fiftieth percentile value is probably not a reasonable standard for the institutionalized elderly patient, since it is based on a healthy and active elderly population. The fifth

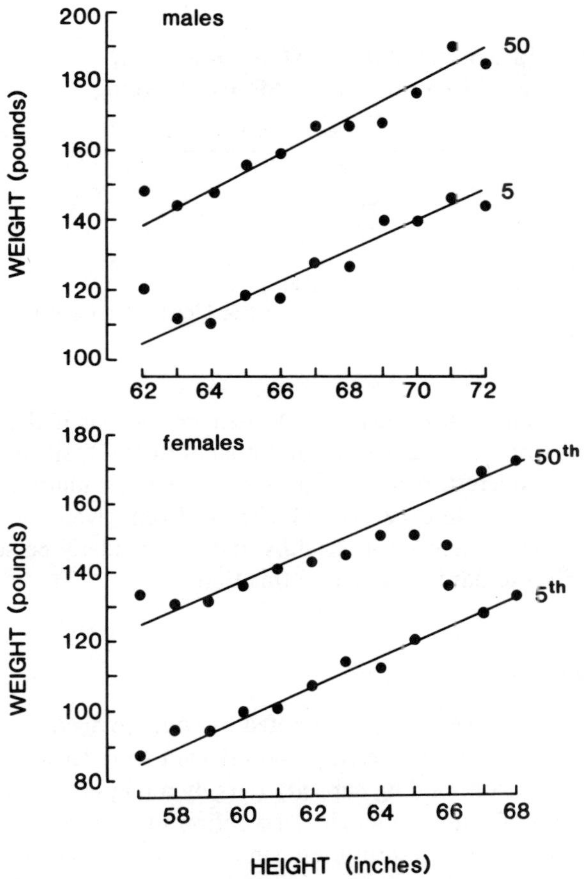

Figure 2-1. Weight of Americans aged 65–74 years, by height, showing the fifth and fiftieth percentiles. Data were derived from the Health and Nutrition Evaluation Survey of 1971–1974 [16].

percentile value could, at least, be used as a minimally acceptable value. Only with further studies, considering relative weight in terms of prognosis, can one say with certainty what is optimal.

Triceps Skinfold and Arm Muscle Circumference. With the previously noted changes in body composition, the standards for these tests need to be re-evaluated for use in the elderly. Table 2-6 gives the fiftieth percentile values from the 1971–1974 HANES survey for women aged 24–34.9 and 65–74.9 years [18]. A possible explanation for why the triceps skinfold (TSF) increases less than one might expect (total body fat is thought to increase by 30 percent) and why arm muscle circumference (AMC) increases rather than decreases

Table 2–6
Changes in Triceps Skinfold (TSF) and Arm Muscle Circumference (AMC) with Aging

Test	*Age*		*Percentage of Change*
	25–34.9	*65–74.9*	
TSF (mm)[a]	21	24	↑14
AMC (cm)[a]	21.2	22.5	↑6

Source: Compiled from Frisancho [18].
[a]Fiftieth percentile values from Health and Nutrition Evaluation Survey of 1971–1974 (females).

(muscle is thought to *decrease* by 40 percent) is that if the compressibility (supporting structure and hydration status) of the fat tissue increases, this will lead to an underestimate of fat and an overestimate of muscle since AMC = arm circumference − (0.134 × TSF). Even given the limitation that these data were gathered from healthy and active elderly persons, they represent the only standard available at this time.

Laboratory Tests

Blood. Albumin levels have been noted by some to decrease with aging [12], but it would be both unnecessary and difficult to redefine the standard. At this time, total iron binding capacity (largely a measure of transferrin) does not change significantly with aging. To define anemia, one should look at the percentage of transferrin saturation, since this is felt to be more accurate than the iron-binding capacity or serum iron levels taken alone [19].

Urine. The 24-hour excretion of creatinine has been the object of much research to date. As noted, the calculation of a patient's creatinine height index is a currently used tool of nutritional assessment. The elderly institutionalized patient will commonly present with a decreased 24-hour urinary creatinine level, and it is important to sort out the relative effects of the three factors that can affect this test value: age, activity status, and nutritional/metabolic status.

Since creatinine is an excellent index of muscle mass, with a documented decreased muscle mass in the elderly one can expect a decrease in creatinine as well. Inactivity will result in further decreases as a result of muscle wasting. Nutritional/metabolic status can also account for decreased creatinine excretion, particularly in marasmic malnutrition. Rowe [20] has documented a decrease in creatinine clearance from 140 ml to 97 ml/min between 30 and 80 years. This documented decline in renal function should not affect the total daily creatinine excretion and, in turn, makes this test less useful in the elderly.

Urinary urea nitrogen (UUN) gives one an excellent index of protein metabolism. Bistrian [2] has utilized the UUN to predict the level of catabolic stress. Increasing levels of stress in a patient will lead to an increase in UUN (indicating catabolism) and a larger discrepancy between the UUN-derived protein intake estimate and the actual protein intake. We have utilized the UUN as a check on the completeness of formula delivery and protein intake [21]. Assuming the patient is in metabolic balance (stable weight, no present stress, infection, or recent surgery), the UUN + 3.5 (a factor for nonurinary urea nitrogen loss—fecal, sweat, integument, and nonurea urinary losses) multiplied by 6.25 (to convert nitrogen to protein) should equal the protein intake. Although there are many factors that can affect the UUN other than dietary nitrogen, this method alerts one to the need to look for complications (including incomplete formula delivery).

Evaluation of Immune Function

Total Lymphocyte Count. The levels of lymphocytes appear not to change with aging to any significant extent [22].

Delayed Hypersensitivity Tests. The response of elderly patients to intradermally placed antigens is an area of current study. Delayed hypersensitivity that is mediated by helper T cells appears to decrease with aging. Studies done using the tuberculin skin test as a measure show a decline in response after age 70 [23]. The impairment appears to involve response not only to previously seen antigens but to new ones as well. Theories explaining these changes focus largely on the phenomenon of thymic involution that occurs with aging. It is the thymus that is the source of T-lymphocytes. If one can expect to see a decreased response to skin tests in the elderly patient, this might lead one away from their use were it not for the fact that these tests come closest to measuring the functional result of poor nutritional status rather than just its presence.

Studies on Chronically Ill, Elderly, Hospitalized Patients

Studies of chronically ill, elderly, hospitalized patients by Dr. A. Palgi of our laboratory have documented that the study population was malnourished in terms of both protein and energy. In these studies of 23 elderly women (mean age 82 years) who were in a chronic care facility due to a variety of chronic medical conditions, nutritional assessment revealed that they were low in weight for height (they averaged 82% of their theoretical ideal based on Metropolitan Life charts, and 86% of the population was less than 85% standard), had a low serum albumin level (average 3.2 g/dl, with 82% of the population less than 3.5 g/dl), and most striking, had a very low 24-hour excretion of urinary creatinine (average 0.44 g/24 hr, which is 54% of the excretion of healthy elderly subjects studied at the Massachusetts Institute of Technology).

As discussed earlier, the correct interpretation of these data depends on whether appropriate standards were used. What is clear is that further work must be done in this area. Since the weight for height is reduced one might suggest high calorie supplementation, but modifications need to be made in light of the urinary creatinine data, which suggest a decrease of 50 percent in muscle mass in these patients. Clearly, replacing this lean body mass with body fat is not the answer.

Further studies on the same population examined the differences in nutritional status between those patients who lived versus those who died. Serum albumin and urinary creatinine levels were found to differ (albumin: 3.23 g/dl in those still living versus 3.04 g/dl in those who later died; creatinine: 0.46 g/24 hr in those still living versus 0.39 g/24 hr in those who later died).

Interpretation of studies of this kind depends on the realization that chronically ill, institutionalized elderly patients present with three overlapping conditions which need to be examined: they are ill, institutionalized (and, most likely, immobilized), and elderly. To begin to sort out the factor of activity level, we compared our patient parameters to those found in free-living (and assumed active) elderly persons. Definite differences were found. In terms of serum albumin levels, for example, while our population had an average value of 3.2 g/dl, free-living elderly studied at MIT had a mean value of 4.2 g/dl. In looking at the illness factor, we compared the albumin levels of our chronically ill elderly to those of acutely ill elderly patients. The acutely ill patients had a mean albumin value of 2.9 g/dl versus our chronically ill patients' value of 3.2 g/dl, which demonstrates the effect of metabolic stress on serum albumin. As already reported, a urinary creatinine level of 0.81 g/24 hr was found in the free-living elderly compared to our population's value of 0.44 g/24 hr. Future studies need to examine further the factor of inactivity in the presence and absence of advanced age and illness, perhaps looking at the creatinine excretion of young motor vehicle accident victims who are completely inactive, young, and usually healthy.

Prognosis

The prognostic power of nutritional assessment parameters has become an active area of research. Harvey [24] examined a variety of assessment parameters and concluded that indeed many have prognostic power. A discriminant function equation for predicting survival based on serum albumin (Alb), reactivity to skin antigen tests for delayed hypersensitivity (DH), and age was 0.96 (Alb) − 1.08 (DH) − 0.02 (age) − 0.22. The overall predictive value was 68.1 percent, sensitivity 69.4 percent, and specificity 64.3 percent. In this acutely ill, hospitalized population, 80 percent of those patients predicted to survive did survive and 40 percent of those predicted to die did die. In the group predicted to die who did not die, improvement in skin antigen testing occurred with conversion from negative to positive recall to *Candida* and mumps antigen tests; thus an improvement in the prognostic index also occurred.

More extensive analysis, in which a larger number of indices were examined, led to the formulation of the Hospital Prognostic Index [24]. Here albumin, delayed hypersensitivity, presence of sepsis, and a diagnosis of cancer were examined and the equation −0.91 (Alb) − 1.00 (DH) − 1.44 (sepsis) + 0.98 (diagnosis) − 1.09 was found to have an overall predictive value for mortality of 72 percent. Albumin taken alone had great power in predicting the probability of energy, sepsis, and death (see Table 2-7).

Few studies of this kind have been conducted specifically in elderly patients. Hodkinson [25] at Hammersmith Hospital, London, examined admission laboratory data and found an overall predictability of survival in a strictly elderly population of 77 percent for men with use of serum Na^+, blood urea nitrogen, T_3 uptake, and hemoglobin, and 84 percent for women with use of these four parameters plus glucose and serum albumin.

Summary

The nutritional assessment of the elderly institutionalized patient is both a challenging and a valuable pursuit. Astute assessment depends on a knowledge of three factors: (1) the assessment parameters in current use, (2) the effects of aging on nutritional status, and (3) the effects of inactivity on nutri-

Table 2–7
Probability Estimates for the Occurrence of Degenerative Processes, Using Serum Albumin Concentrations

Degenerative Process	*Serum Albumin Concentration (g/dl) at Indicated Probabilities*				
	< 0.10	*< 0.25*	*0.50*	*> 0.75*	*> 0.90*
Anergy	5.2	4.2	3.2	2.2	1.2
Sepsis	4.3	3.7	3.1	2.5	1.9
Death	4.9	4.0	3.2	2.3	1.5

Source: Compiled from Harvey et al. [24].

tional status. Specifically, one must consider the effects of aging on the nutritional assessment parameters being utilized. These topics have been discussed here, and we have presented some recent data from our laboratory on the nutritional assessment of chronically ill, elderly hospitalized patients and the prognostic power of nutritional assessment data. Despite the limitations pointed out in terms of the current absence of age-specific tests and standards, we must continue to gather the necessary data for the formulation of appropriate standards in order to provide better care for this very special population group.

References

1. Blackburn, G.L., Bistrian, B.R., Maini, B.S., et al. Nutritional and metabolic assessment of the hospitalized patient. *J.P.E.N.* 1:11–22, 1977.

2. Bistrian, B.R. A simple technique to estimate the severity of stress. *Surg. Gynecol. Obstet.* 148:675–678, 1979.

3. Forbes, G.B., Bruining, G.J. Urinary creatinine excretion and lean body mass. *Am. J. Clin. Nutr.* 29:1359–1366, 1976.

4. Bistrian, B.R., Blackburn, G.L., Sherman, M., Scrimshaw, N.S. Therapeutic index of nutritional depletion in hospitalized patients. *Surg. Gynecol. Obstet.* 141:512–516, 1975.

5. Munro, H.N. Nutrition and aging. *Br. Med. J.* 37:83–88, 1981.

6. Forbes, G.B. The adult decline in lean body mass. *Hum. Biol.* 48:161–173, 1976.

7. Korenchevsky, V. *Physiological and Pathological Aging.* Basel: Karger, 1961.

8. Garn, S.M. In Farmer, F.A. (Ed.), *Nutrition of the Aged.* Alberta: University of Calgary, 1978. Pp. 73–90.

9. Gregerman, R.I. In Gitman, L. (Ed.), *Endocrines and Aging.* New York: MSF Information, 1967. Pp. 161–173.

10. Uauy, R., Winterer, J.C., Bilmazes, C., et al. The changing pattern of whole body protein metabolism in aging humans. *J. Gerontol.* 33:663–671, 1978.

11. Munro, H.N., Young, V.R. Urinary excretion of N,t-methylhistidine (3-methylhistidine): A tool to study metabolic responses in relation to nutrient and hormonal status in health and disease of man. *Am. J. Clin. Nutr.* 31:1608–1614, 1978.

12. Gersovitz, M., Munro, H.N., Udall, J., Young, V.R. Albumin synthesis in young and elderly subjects using a new stable isotope methodology: Response to level of protein intake. *Metabolism* 29:1075–1086, 1980.

13. Misra, D.P., Loudon, J.M., Staddon, G.E. Albumin metabolism in elderly patients. *J. Gerontol.* 30:304–306, 1975.

14. Mitchell, C.O., Lipshitz, D.A. Detection of protein-calorie malnutrition in the elderly. *Am. J. Clin. Nutr.* 35:398–406, 1982.

15. Mitchell, C.O., Lipshitz, D.A. Arm length measurement as an alternative to height in nutritional assessment of the elderly. *J.P.E.N.* 6:226–229, 1982.

16. National Center for Health Statistics. *Weight by Height and Age of Adults 18–74 Years: U.S., 1971–1974.* Vital and Health Statistics, ser. 11, no. 208. Washington, D.C.: U.S. Government Printing Office, 1974.

17. Master, A.M., Lasser, R.P., Beckman, G. Tables of average weight and height of Americans aged 65 to 94 years. *J.A.M.A.* 172:114–118, 1960.

18. Frisancho, A.R. New norms of upper limb fat and muscle areas for assessment of nutritional status. *Am. J. Clin. Nutr.* 34:2540–2545, 1981.

19. Awad, M.O., Barford, A.V., Grindulis, K.A., et al. Factors affecting the serum iron-binding capacity in the elderly. *Gerontology* 28:124–131, 1982.

20. Rowe, J.W., Andres, R., Tobin, J.D., et al. The effect of age on creatinine clearance in men. A cross-sectional and longitudinal study. *J. Gerontol.* 31:155–163, 1976.

21. Clark, N.G., Rappaport, J.I., Lamothe, P.A., et al. Use of urinary urea nitrogen excretion to predict protein intakes (abstract). *Age* 5:138, 1982.

22. Sparrow, D., Silbert, J.E., Rowe, J.W. The influence of age on peripheral lymphocyte count in men: A cross-sectional and longitudinal study. *J. Gerontol.* 35:163–166, 1980.

23. Weksler, M.E. The senescence of the immune system. *Hosp. Pract.* 16:53–64, 1981.

24. Harvey, K.B., Moldawer, L.L., Bistrian, B.R., Blackburn, G.L. Biological measures for the formulation of a hospital prognostic index. *Am. J. Clin. Nutr.* 34:2013–2022, 1981.

25. Hodkinson, H.M. Value of admission profile tests for prognosis in elderly patients. *J. Am. Geriatr. Soc.* 29:206–210, 1981.

26. Blackburn, G.L. Nutritional assessment: An overview. In *Clinical Consultations in Nutritional Support*, vol. 1. Chicago: Medical Directions, 1981 P. 10.

3 Special Nutritional Requirements of the Young and the Old

Richard S. Rivlin, M.D.

Each age has its own special nutritional concerns. For the young, proper nutrition is critical to enable normal growth and development to occur. Both obesity and extreme underweight in childhood should be avoided. It is essential to consider the special nutritional requirements of young people in two particular situations where the knowledge and advice of health professionals may be vital, namely anorexia nervosa and extreme vegetarianism. In anorexia nervosa and its variants, there may be severe malnutrition, high morbidity, and complex metabolic changes occurring as a result of the extreme weight loss. In extreme vegetarianism, strict followers of this practice may be at risk for developing deficiencies of certain specific nutrients, as well as of total calories. Anorexia nervosa and vegetarianism deserve special consideration because both are not rare and are possibly increasing in prevalence in the United States at the present time.

Special Concerns of the Young

It is essential that health practitioners be aware of the early manifestations of anorexia nervosa in young people so that proper consideration can be given to the serious nature of this psychiatric disorder. Knowledge of vegetarianism and its ramifications is also essential in order that appropriate nutritional guidance can be given to vegetarians, a matter of particular concern during pregnancy.

Anorexia Nervosa

It does not usually require great clinical acumen to diagnose anorexia nervosa in an advanced stage; there may be enormous degrees of malnutrition and

This work was supported by NIH grants 5P01 CA-29502, IT32 CA-09427 and NCI-CM-15735, and by grants from the Stella and Charles Guttman Foundation, the National Dairy Council, the National Live Stock and Meat Board, the William H. Donner Foundation, the United States Brewers Association, the Fairchild Foundation, the Richard Molin Foundation, Hoffmann-LaRoche Inc., the General Foods Fund, and the Velmans Fund. The research was performed in the Sperry Corporation Nutrition Research Laboratory.

Table 3-1
Criteria for Diagnosis of Anorexia Nervosa

Age of onset prior to 25
Weight loss of at least 25% of original body weight
Distorted attitudes toward eating, food, or body weight (e.g., denial, enjoying food refusal, desire to be extremely thin)
No known medical illness
No known psychiatric disorder
At least two of the following:
amenorrhea
lanugo hair
bradycardia
periods of overactivity
episodes of gorging
vomiting

Source: Adapted from Feighner et al [1].

wasting and very obvious personality patterns. The challenge is to detect this disorder at an early stage. Although anorexia nervosa is usually associated with white middle-class and upper-class young women, its incidence in other racial and ethnic groups has increased in conjunction with the increased upward socioeconomic mobility of these groups. Finding a child with anorexia nervosa in a family may, in fact, be an indication that the family has "arrived" at a higher social level.

The classic criteria for the diagnosis of anorexia nervosa are shown in Table 3-1 [1]. The age of onset is characteristically during adolescence, but late onset occasionally occurs and often carries a poor prognosis. Weight loss of at least 25 percent of original body weight certainly will produce many metabolic changes, but these often develop with much lower amounts of weight loss. Distorted attitudes toward eating occur frequently in the adolescent population, and health professionals must be able to distinguish between typical behavior and signs of a more severe underlying disturbance. Typically, there is no other known medical or psychiatric disorder. Certain findings on history or features on physical examination deserve special mention in this context. Amenorrhea is of course the classic manifestation of this condition, and may be one of a number of complex hypothalamic-pituitary disturbances that are present. Lanugo hair, similar to that in young infants, is often apparent, particularly on the back and extremities.

The occurrence of periods of overactivity, sometimes compulsive, is a feature of the disorder that does not receive sufficient attention by health professionals. In some instances the weight loss may be meaningfully related more to the increased energy expenditure than to the reduced energy intake, and this feature may be more readily susceptible to treatment. Patients may

Table 3–2
Some Features of Anorexia Nervosa

Incidence probably 0.4 to 1.0% of age group
Patients generally middle- and upper-class with well-educated parents
Family history of anorexia nervosa and obesity
Weight loss initiated by dieting
Morbid fear of gaining weight
Denial of thinness; distorted body image
Preoccupation with food
Lack of sexual interest
Hypothermia
Sleep disturbances and depression
High incidence of complications in pregnancy and delivery
Premorbid personality: well-behaved, perfectionistic, competitive, achieving
Hypotension and functional heart murmurs
Chronic constipation
Death rate approximately 5% overall

be better able to accept a philosophy of "ride, don't walk" and "take it easy" than they are to accept close supervision of every mouthful of food eaten.

Other features of anorexia nervosa, summarized in Table 3-2, are largely self-evident. Historical details such as gorging and vomiting are important to elicit, as they may be indicative of a serious personality disturbance. It is essential to know the family situation and the interpersonal dynamics; curiously, both anorexia nervosa and obesity tend to be familial and both may occur in the same family. Health professionals should realize that anorexia nervosa is not rare and carries a significant overall mortality rate. The hypothermia, reduced body fat, and overactivity may pose real risks for these patients in the winter when they are subjected to cold exposure.

The major nutritional requirements in anorexia nervosa can be summarized simply as consuming more food of good quality and burning up fewer calories. These objectives are often difficult to achieve and require a team of health professionals including an internist or pediatrician, psychiatrist, and dietitian. It is discouraging that the results of treatment are often poor, relapses occur frequently, and the condition is often of prolonged duration [2].

Vegetarianism

In general, vegetarianism is compatible with a long, healthy life provided there is sufficient diversification in the diet and adequate calorie intake is

Table 3-3
Classification of Vegetarians

Class	*Food Consumed*
Lactoovovegetarians	No meat; consume vegetables, dairy products and eggs
Lactovegetarians	No meat or eggs; consume vegetables and dairy products
Fruitarians	No meat, eggs, or dairy products; consume only raw or dried fruits or nuts
Vegans	No animal or dairy products

Source: Derived from data published by the National Dairy Council [3].

maintained. The main problem with vegetarianism is the limited diet and selection. Since protein from animal sources is usually of somewhat higher quality than that from plant sources, it is necessary to vary the plant sources of protein to be certain that all the essential amino acids have been ingested in adequate quantities. For example, cereal grains generally tend to have a relatively low level of lysine, while beans and peas have adequate levels of lysine but are relatively deficient in methionine. A diet containing all these foods would more likely be nutritionally complete [3,4].

The generally accepted classification of vegetarians is given in Table 3-3. The degree to which individuals are potentially at risk for a deficiency of a particular nutrient likely depends both on the duration of following vegetarian practices and on the strictness of adherence. Thus, of the groups examined, vegans are most likely to develop deficiencies [3].

There are at least five major nutrients for which there is a potential for developing deficiencies in vegetarianism: vitamin B_{12}, vitamin B_2 (riboflavin), calcium, iron, and zinc. It is well known that vitamin B_{12} can only be obtained from animal sources, and therefore one would expect deficiency to develop frequently in vegetarians. However, frank vitamin B_{12} deficiency is actually relatively uncommon in vegans, probably for several reasons. First, small amounts of vitamin B_{12} manage to creep into the diet from unexpected sources. Seaweed, a common item among certain vegetarian groups, contains a great deal of vitamin B_{12}. Second, since it takes a number of years to deplete body sources of vitamin B_{12} to the deficiency level, many individuals may not be following the dietary practices long enough to be at risk.

Riboflavin is present in the American diet in largest amounts in meat and meat products, and in milk and dairy products. Most dietary surveys reveal that riboflavin intake will be adequate provided there is sufficient meat and milk in the diet. If riboflavin is to be consumed from vegetarian sources only, large amounts of the vegetables must be eaten to meet these needs. Furthermore, the methods of food preparation are important. Riboflavin is both light-sensitive and alkali-sensitive. The addition of baking soda to green vegetables, a practice that is done to preserve color, may result in considerable loss of biological activity. Although definitive data are not currently available, it is extremely likely that sun drying of fruits and vegetables causes considerable loss of the riboflavin content [5].

Calcium, iron, and zinc may not be contained in large amounts in vegetable sources, and data are accumulating to suggest that they may be somewhat less bioavailable. The increasing use of high-fiber diets raises the possibility that these metals may not be absorbed in adequate quantities, but the clinical significance of these observations requires further study. The recent findings that tea may inhibit iron absorption and vitamin C enhances iron absorption from nonheme sources indicate how common food items may interact with one another and influence nutritional status.

The greatest potential difficulties with vegetarian practices may arise when they are strict, prolonged, and nondiversified and when they involve pregnancy and childhood [6]. It may be difficult for vegetarians to maintain adequate caloric intake during pregnancy and childhood, and the disturbing reports of rickets and of developmental problems in offspring of vegetarian mothers are of serious concern to health professionals. Vegetarianism is not confined to young people, and these considerations will apply to older people as well, in whom the consequences of calcium deficiency in particular may be especially meaningful.

Special Concerns of the Elderly

At the older end of the age scale, many important physiologic changes have occurred in a process that has been evolving over one's lifetime. Many functions have declined since young adulthood. The nutritional requirements of the elderly are beginning to attract attention as we recognize that this segment is growing faster than any other segment of the population, is often isolated and impoverished, and may be in marginal nutritional status. The elderly as a group are most at risk for developing drug-induced nutritional deficiencies because of their prolonged use of drugs, their dependence on multiple drugs, and their compromised nutritional status.

Physiologic Changes with Aging

In considering the nutritional needs of the elderly, it is essential to recall that body composition and metabolism change fundamentally with aging. Older people are fatter in the sense that they have a relatively high proportion of body fat to lean body mass compared to their younger counterparts. This finding is likely to be a result of both an accumulation of fat tissue and an actual decline in lean body mass [7]. It is well known that the rate of protein synthesis decreases with aging, and that many anabolic processes generally decrease in older people.

In view of the relative decrease in lean body mass with aging, it is not surprising that there also occurs a decrease in the metabolic rate [8]. Muscle mass contributes to metabolic rate more than does any other tissue, and the age-related decline in muscle tissue would be expected to result in a reduction in the metabolic rate. An important question to answer is whether the changes in body composition are sufficient in magnitude to account for this reduction in oxygen consumption. A diminution in thyroid function with aging could also contribute to the reduced metabolic rate, but those changes in thyroid parameters that have been observed with aging are not particularly impressive [9].

Fascinating longitudinal studies in rats suggest that the magnitude of the lean body mass in young adults may have prognostic value in terms of longevity and health. There appears to be a natural selection process that occurs with aging, resulting in more prolonged survival of those animals that have a relatively small lean body mass to begin with in early adulthood [10]. Thus, some loss of lean body mass undoubtedly occurs with aging, but this may be only part of the picture; the ability of animals with a small lean body mass earlier in life to prevail as old age approaches may also be critical.

In addition to these overall changes, nutritional status is dependent on specific physiologic changes that occur with aging. Important physiologic factors that may modify nutritional status in the elderly include decreased ability to taste and smell, loss of teeth, decreased gastric acidity, reduced secretion of intestinal enzymes, malabsorption, and decreased hepatic and renal function.

A useful concept applicable to understanding the problems of the elderly, and one that is particularly relevant to the field of nutrition, is that of sensory deprivation [11]. By living alone and eating alone, as all too many of our elderly do, they are deprived of stimulating contacts and interactions with other human beings. Physiologically, the progressive loss of vision is a critical aspect of sensory deprivation. Much is written about the need for more detailed and informative nutritional labeling of food items, but the advances that have been made already are of little benefit to elderly people if they cannot read the labels. A service program of providing teenage escorts for the urban elderly when they go shopping is reassuring in terms of protection against possible assault, but it may serve an even more valuable function by helping the elderly to read labels in the stores. Cooking is a hazard for elderly people with impaired vision, and the possibility of their starting fires or receiving scalds or burns is an ever-present danger.

Loss of hearing also results in progressive removal of the elderly from the mainstream of life. Unfortunately, reduced hearing is often treated with ridicule rather than with understanding by many younger people. It has been speculated that the sound of food in the mouth is a factor leading to its enjoyment, and one of which the elderly are deprived.

More recent is the recognition that loss of ability to taste and smell may be a feature of aging [12,13]. Defects occur not only for the tastes of pure solutions but particularly of common food items. Elderly people frequently comment that food items taste weak or bland to them, and they may use higher concentrations of condiments in order to give food items their customary taste. This tendency may result in excessive salting of food, an obvious hazard to patients with congestive heart failure, and may possibly lead to hypertension in susceptible individuals if this practice is continued over a prolonged period. The inability to distinguish rancid food from unspoiled food, which probably involves sensations of smell more than of taste, poses the potential risk of severe food poisoning. The frequent observation that serious fires in apartment buildings result in the death of a disproportionate number of elderly inhabitants is usually attributed to their lack of agility in removing themselves from the building. One cannot help wondering, in the light of recent documentation of impaired sensory status, whether a more significant factor may be that the elderly simply cannot smell the smoke. Diminished taste and smell sensations in older people not only may present risks to them, but more fundamentally, may result in less enjoyment of food, less enthusiasm about eating, and more limited food selection. More research is needed on sensory function in the elderly.

Nutrition and Cancer

Cancer is to some extent a disease of aging, and the accumulated evidence to date suggests that nutritional factors may be relevant to the cause of certain cancers, such as those of the breast, colon, and prostate. Although it is still a subject of great controversy, the bulk of the evidence to date from both animal and human studies supports the hypothesis that the total amount of fat in the diet, and perhaps also the degree of saturation, may be factors in tumor development [14].

With respect to these cancers, there are strong positive correlations between dietary fat consumption and the prevalence of these tumors in various nations. In Thailand and El Salvador, breast cancer is practically unknown; whether this low prevalence is due entirely to low dietary fat intake is unlikely, but it is very clear that these countries have among the lowest average fat intakes known. By contrast, in the Netherlands and in Denmark, where dietary fat intake is enormous, the prevalence of breast cancer is also very high [15]. Generally similar relationships pertain to colon and prostate cancer. There are, of course, important genetic relationships also; Greece has about the same average dietary fat intake as Israel, but only one-third the prevalence of breast cancer.

The mechanisms relating intake of dietary fat to cancer promotion are no doubt complex and may involve changes in the rates of formation of secondary bile acids, alterations in the flora of the intestinal tract, enhanced

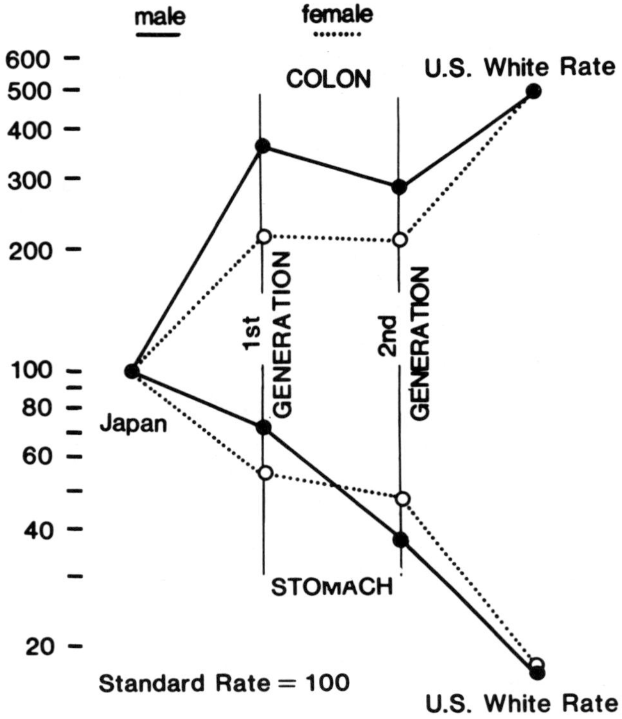

Figure 3-1. Relative mortality rates from colon and stomach cancer among Japanese migrants of both sexes to the United States, as compared with the mortality rate among native Japanese and natives of the United States (Caucasian race). Data were derived from Haenszel and Kurihara [17].

rates of drug metabolism, alteration of sex hormone production, and other mechanisms as well. But striking evidence for environmental effects as important factors in cancer prevalence comes from a frequently cited study showing that Japanese who migrate to the United States and Hawaii undergo changes in prevalence of cancer of the colon and stomach which are in the direction of the native United States population. Thus, as shown in Figure 3-1, the risk of colon cancer increases and that of stomach cancer decreases after migration to the United States. These changes were demonstrable in the first generation of migrants [16,17]. These studies do not prove that the environmental factor was diet, however, and further research is needed to exclude other influences.

Studies involving dietary fat are only one example of the broad range of studies now in progress to evaluate the effect of a single dietary nutrient, such as vitamin A, vitamin C, riboflavin, alcohol, and others [18]. Critical research remains to be done to extend the findings in experimental animals to man, and to perform the necessary intervention studies with specific nutrients. The nutritional requirements of the elderly population must be considered in light of the fact that dietary practices may influence the development of both cardiovascular disease and cancer. It is likely that the maximum benefit to be derived from dietary factors may depend on prolonged periods of time in which they are at work. Thus the nutritional requirements of the young must be considered in terms of their long-range consequences, and the nutritional research must be directed at both the young and the old [19].

Summary

Special nutritional requirements are highlighted in the young and elderly population. In young people, anorexia nervosa and strict vegetarianism are of particular concern.

Early detection of anorexia nervosa goes far in the successful treatment of this serious psychiatric disorder. Even though this condition is not rare and carries a high mortality rate, it is not easily recognized early by clinicians. The objectives of treatment, consuming more and burning up less, are best achieved by a team approach including an internist or pediatrician, psychiatrist, and dietitian. Nevertheless, the results are often discouraging and the prognosis for these patients is frequently poor.

In general, vegetarianism is compatible with a long, healthy life provided there is sufficient diversification in the diet and adequate caloric intake is maintained. Lack of vitamin B_{12}, vitamin B_2, calcium, iron, and zinc represents the most likely nutritional deficiencies in vegetarians, and such potential lack is most serious during childhood, pregnancy, and old age.

The recognition that body composition, metabolism, and nutritional needs change with age has only come recently. Partly for this reason, increasing emphasis from a nutritionist's viewpoint has been focused on the elderly. Both cancer and cardiovascular disease are mainly associated with the elderly, and they have shown a strong link with lifelong dietary practices. Numerous studies are in progress to evaluate the effect of several single dietary constituents on the nutritional requirements and health of the elderly.

References

1. Feighner, J.P. Robins, E., Guze, S.B., et al. Diagnostic criteria for use in psychiatric research. *Arch. Gen. Psychiatry* 26:57–63, 1972.

2. Vigersky, R. (Ed.). *Anorexia Nervosa*. New York: Raven Press, 1977.

3. National Dairy Council. Nutrition and vegetarianism. *Dairy Council Digest* 50:1–5, 1979.

4. Crosby, W.H. Can a vegetarian be well nourished? *J.A.M.A.* 233:898, 1975.

5. Hunt, S.H. Nutritional intake of riboflavin. In Rivlin, R.S. (Ed.), *Riboflavin.* New York: Plenum Press, 1975. Pp. 199–219.

6. Dwyer, J.T., Dietz, W.H., Hass, G., Suskind, R. Risk of nutritional rickets among vegetarian children. *Am. J. Dis. Child.* 133:134–140, 1979.

7. Pierson, R.H., Jr., Lin, D.H.Y., Phillips, R.A. Total body potassium in health: Effects of age, sex, height and fat. *Am. J. Physiol.* 226:206–212, 1974.

8. Shock, N.W. Metabolism and age (review). *J. Chronic Dis.* 2:687–703, 1955.

9. Gregerman, R.I., Bierman, E.L. Aging and hormones. In Williams, R.H. (Ed.), *Textbook of Endocrinology*, 5th ed. Philadelphia: W.B. Saunders, 1974. Pp. 1059–1070.

10. Lesser, G.T., Deutsch, S., Markofsky, J. Aging in the rat: Longitudinal and cross-sectional studies of body composition. *Am. J. Physiol.* 225:1472–1478, 1973.

11. Rivlin, R.S. Nutrition and aging: Some unanswered questions. *Am. J. Med.* 71:337–340, 1981.

12. Cooper, R.M., Bilach, I., Zubek, J.P. The effect of age on taste sensitivity. *J. Gerontol.* 14:56–58, 1959.

13. Schiffman, S. Food recognition by the elderly. *J. Gerontol.* 32:586–592, 1977.

14. Newell, G.R., Ellison, N.M. (Eds.). *Nutrition and Cancer: Etiology and Treatment.* New York: Raven Press, 1981.

15. Reddy, B.S., Cohen, L.A., McCoy, G.D., et al. Nutrition and its relationship to cancer. *Adv. Cancer Res.* 32:237–345, 1980.

16. Haenszel, W.M., Berg, J.W., Segi, M., et al. Large bowel cancer in Hawaiian Japanese. *J. Natl. Cancer Inst.* 51:401–414, 1975.

17. Haenszel, W.M., Kurihara, M. Studies of Japanese migrants: I. Mortality from cancer and other diseases among Japanese in the United States. *J. Natl. Cancer Inst.* 40:43–68, 1968.

18. Rivlin, R.S. Nutrition and cancer: State of the art. Relationship of several nutrients to the development of cancer. *J. Am. Coll. Nutr.* 1:75–88, 1982.

19. Rivlin, R.S., Young, E.A. (Eds.). Symposium on evidence relating selected vitamins and minerals to health and disease in the elderly population in the United States. *Am. J. Clin. Nutr.* (Suppl.) 36:977–1086, 1982.

Discussion

Questions were presented by the audience to the panel of speakers: Dr. Hodges, Mr. Clark, and Dr. Rivlin.

The panel and the audience entered into a lively discussion over the inadequacy of the current height/weight tables as a nutritional assessment tool. It was pointed out that particularly in elderly patients, accurate height measurements are difficult to obtain. Furthermore, sedentary behavior may lead to conditions that decrease height, and certain disease states such as lower limb contracture and osteoporosis make it difficult to measure height accurately. In the latter instances, it was suggested that body length could be approximated by the use of a flexible tape measure following body contour; alternatively, long bone length has been suggested as an index of body height and serum creatinine levels as an index of lean body mass.

Whereas it may be possible to determine accurately body weight measurements in the elderly, Mr. Clark commented that if obesity is regarded as a health risk factor per se, then as the population grows older the survivors will be lean. He was quick to point out, however, that such a conclusion may be based on static, cross-sectional data rather than on longitudinal data. Further, he added, the individual at 100 to 125 percent of "ideal" weight is in a slightly better position prognostically than one who is slightly below ideal weight if the latter is a heavy smoker and if he is underweight due to early illness. Dr. Hodges added that obesity per se does not appear to be an independent risk factor (in terms of life expectancy) in the absence of diabetes, hypertension, and hyperlipidemia. In the final analysis, it was agreed that the present height/weight tables may not be directly applicable to the elderly and that body weight in slight excess of "ideal" would probably be acceptable. Clearly, more research is needed on this important subject.

On the other hand, it must be recognized that chronic inactivity will lead to a decrease in muscle mass and a relative increase in the proportion of body fat. Measurement of urinary creatinine excretion may be a more useful tool than body weight in nutritional assessment. Indeed, the muscle mass of an individual is a function of four distinct factors: nutritional status, medical status, activity status, and age. Separation of one of these from the other three may lead to fallacious conclusions. In this regard it must be pointed out that very little is known about the nutritional needs of completely inactive patients at any age. There is no doubt that continuing exercise and physical activity throughout life have beneficial, stimulatory effects on the musculoskeletal system.

The issue of mineral and vitamin requirements and supplements raised considerable discussion. Adequate calcium intake in both the young and the elderly was given very high priority for normal bone elongation in the former and bone renewal in the latter. Adequate calcium supply can be assured through sufficient intake of milk and dairy products.

This discussion raised the question of lactose intolerance. Dr. Rivlin pointed out that true lactose intolerance must be established diagnostically rather than merely suspected before it is treated. In this regard, it must be recognized that chronic malnutrition leads to atrophy of the intestinal villi.

Villous atrophy, in turn, results in loss of intestinal lactase, which is the cause of lactose intolerance. Even very brief periods of malnutrition may cause some degree of lactose intolerance. However, this condition is reversible, and it is possible to return a patient to a normal diet eventually.

Several alternatives are available to people who have lactose intolerance. Often such individuals will tolerate small quantities of milk at several different times during a day. They can also try chocolate milk, which is often tolerated better by lactose-intolerant persons than is regular milk. A commercially available product called LactAid, which contains lactase, can be used to treat the milk before its use. It should also be pointed out that certain cheeses produced by bacterial action (e.g., hard cheese, yogurt without additives) are an excellent source of calcium because the bacteria cleave the lactose molecule. If these possibilities are exhausted, use of calcium supplements should be instituted. Supplementation may be accomplished by oral administration of various calcium salts such as calcium lactate, calcium gluconate, or calcium carbonate. Of these, calcium carbonate is probably preferable since it contains the highest amount of calcium by weight and is also the least expensive. As much as 2.5 g/day of elemental calcium can be given in this manner without the risk of calcium toxicity, according to Dr. Heaney and his colleagues at the University of Nebraska. (TUMS antacid tablets contain 500 mg of $CaCO_3$.)

The question of teratogenicity of megadoses of vitamins (A, B, C, D) during pregnancy was raised by the audience. The panel agreed that some objective data are available on this issue, but much evidence is still anecdotal. In pregnant rats, massive doses of vitamin C tended either to produce teratogenic effects or to lead to spontaneous abortion. Hypercalcemia in pregnant women, which can result from overdosage of vitamin D, is thought to result in cardiac and other malformations in the offspring. Some clinical studies have suggested that large doses of vitamin A appear to be teratogenic in humans. On the other hand, in one study, women given multiple-vitamin preparations tended to have some protection against the likelihood of delivering a child that was deformed—at least in terms of neural tube defects. In this study, the doses were in the range of recommended daily allowances rather than in megadose proportions. More research is needed on the pros and cons of vitamin supplementation during pregnancy.

The panel agreed that there is little reason for giving vitamin supplements to healthy children. If children are well-nourished, they probably do not need these supplements. Only if eating is very erratic should vitamin supplementation be considered. One population in whom such action might be taken, as Dr. Hodges pointed out, are children, especially teenagers, who generally skip breakfast and eat most of their meals outside the home.

The panel was questioned on the use of salt (NaCl) in the diet, especially in regard to a salt-restricted diet. Agreement was unanimous that moderate salt restriction would not usually lead to malnutrition. From a dietitian's point of view, many spices can be substituted for salt to make food tasty. Furthermore, Dr. Rivlin added an important comment concerning the physiology of taste: The ability to taste saltiness is the result of differences between the concentration of NaCl in food and in saliva; only if the salt concentration in food is higher than that in saliva does the food have a salty taste. As less salt is added to food, less will be excreted in the saliva, and eventually less salt will be required in food to achieve a salty taste. After a period of adjustment, patients on a low-salt diet often find that it is less bland than when they first started it, perhaps because of this phenomenon.

In addressing the problem of anorexia nervosa, members of the panel pointed out that there exists no known correlation between this disorder and alcohol or drug dependence. Vegetarianism is not regarded as a "safe" substitute for or variant of anorexia. People do not usually develop anorexia nervosa out of fear of certain types of food but more out of fear of excess calories and perceived fatness. In males, anorexia nervosa is not common but has a very poor prognosis, perhaps because it is not recognized until very late.

Rehabilitation of the malnourished patient was discussed at some length. It was agreed that it is of primary importance to evaluate the patient's height/weight ratio. Serum albumin levels were not regarded as a good indicator of nutritional status, despite being a function of a host of different factors. Moreover, their use as a rehabilitative measure is limited by a long half-life of 18 to 20 days. It is important to be cognizant of the patient's lean body mass as related to his physical activity level. Therefore, a measure of lean body mass, such as serum creatinine concentration, may be more appropriate. It is important to recognize that increased caloric feeding of the inactive patient may result in fat deposition. Thus, it is important not to overfeed the chronically bedridden, inactive patient.

II Nutrition in Health and Disease

4 The Vitamin D Endocrine System in Health and Disease

Hector F. DeLuca, Ph.D.

In 1919 Sir Edward Mellanby successfully produced the disease rickets in dogs by feeding them a diet of oatmeal and housing them indoors. This disease, which was quite similar to the then rampant disease in the human population, could be cured or prevented by the administration of cod liver oil [1]. Since cod liver oil had been demonstrated by McCollum to contain a fat-soluble vitamin A, it was the conclusion of Sir Edward Mellanby that the healing of rickets was another property of fat-soluble vitamin A. McCollum and his colleagues, however, quickly recognized that this antirachitic activity was distinct from the growth-promoting and antixerophthalmic activity that McCollum and Davis had discovered earlier in the cod liver oil. By bubbling oxygen through cod liver oil and heating it, they could destroy the vitamin A activity but retain the ability to heal rickets [2]. McCollum concluded, therefore, that this represented a new vitamin, which he termed "fat-soluble vitamin D."

While the discoveries of Sir Edward Mellanby were taking place, a Viennese physician was able to show that sunlight or artificial ultraviolet light could also heal rickets [3]. Thus it appeared that cod liver oil and ultraviolet light had equal biologic activity. This dilemma was solved when Steenbock demonstrated that ultraviolet light could induce, in the lipid fractions of food and skin, the presence of the antirachitic substance [4]. Since food could be irradiated with ultraviolet light, it became simple to eliminate rickets as a major medical problem by merely inducing vitamin D in some foods by irradiation. Furthermore, the discovery of irradiation of the plant and animal sterols with ultraviolet light to produce vitamin D led to the isolation and chemical identification of vitamin D in 1932 [5]. This reached its conclusion in 1937 when Windaus and his colleagues isolated and identified vitamin D_3 [6]. The structure of this form of vitamin D is shown in Figure 4-1, since it illustrates the natural form of vitamn D that is normally produced in skin with ultraviolet irradiation. In addition to this form of vitamin D, another form is produced by the irradiation of the plant sterol, ergosterol. This other form, vitamin D_2, differs from vitamin D_3 in the structure of the side chain (Fig. 4-1). Both compounds are equally effective in man, as is currently known.

This work was supported by Program Project Grant AM-14881 from the National Institutes of Health and by the Harry Steenbock Research Fund of the Wisconsin Alumni Research Foundation.

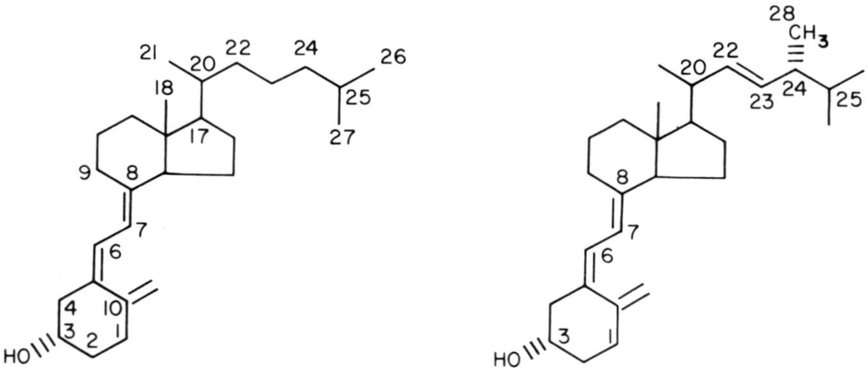

Vitamin D_3 Vitamin D_2

Figure 4-1. Structures of the two main nutritional forms of vitamin D including their numbering system.

Vitamin D is in reality not a vitamin, since it can be normally photobiosynthesized in skin. In recent years some progress has been made in our understanding of the biogenesis of vitamin D in skin. It is now quite clear that 7-dehydrocholesterol, a compound in abundance in skin as an intermediate in cholesterol biosynthesis, undergoes a strictly chemical photolysis reaction in the epidermis to yield a substance called "previtamin D_3," as shown in Figure 4-2 [7,8]. Previtamin D is by itself either biologically inactive or very much less active than vitamin D itself. This compound is in equilibrium with vitamin D_3, as Figure 4-2 shows. At body temperature this equilibration requires approximately 36 hours to complete [9]. Of considerable interest is the fact that previtamin D_3 does not leave the skin, since it is not recognized by the vitamin D transport protein in the plasma [9]. However, as it slowly equilibrates to form vitamin D_3, the vitamin D_3 is transferred from the skin to the plasma bound to the vitamin D transport globulin, a protein of 52,000 molecular weight [10]. The photolysis of 7-dehydrocholesterol in skin appears to be a strictly chemical reaction that is identical with the same reaction known to occur in organic solvents; it does not appear to be a biologically controlled reaction [7,8]. The fact that vitamin D_3 is made in skin then requires the view that vitamin D is a dietary requirement only because man does not expose himself to sufficient amounts of ultraviolet light. Fortunately, vitamin D can be absorbed with the fats in the distal small intestine through the lacteal system into the chylomicrons and subsequently is cleared by the liver. Vitamin D produced in skin is also delivered to the liver, where this compound accumulates in a rather specific manner [11].

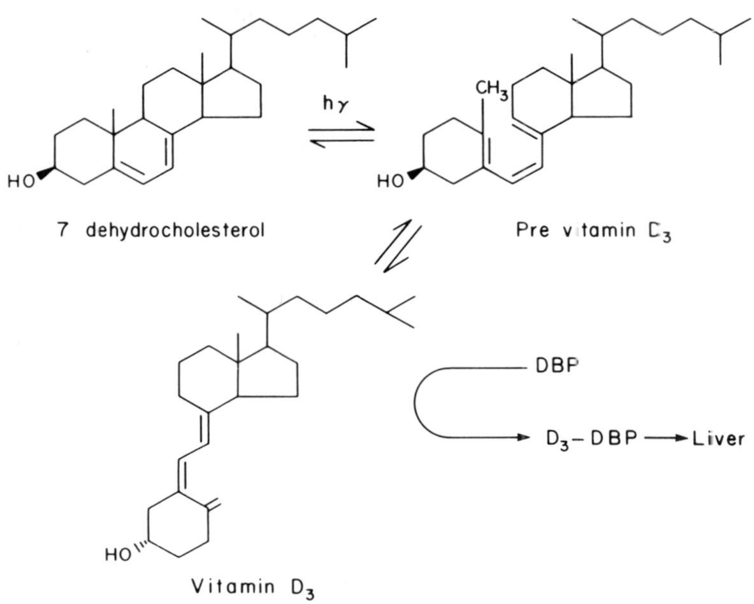

Figure 4-2. Structural representation of the photobiogenesis of vitamin D in epidermis. Note that the previtamin D is the obligatory intermediate but is retained in the skin since it is not transported via the vitamin D transport protein (DBP).

There is inadequate information available concerning the efficiency of production of vitamin D in skin, although it now appears that it is an efficient process in which exposure of approximately 10 percent of the body to summer sunlight for 10 minutes is sufficient to produce adequate amounts of vitamin D to meet the needs of the organism [12].

Functions of Vitamin D

Vitamin D is known to prevent or heal three disorders. First, it plays an important function in correcting hypocalcemia, a function it shares with the parathyroid hormone [13,14]. A second important physiologic function is to prevent the disease rickets in the young [1]; a third is to prevent osteomalacia in the adult [15]. Rickets and osteomalacia are very closely related disorders. Both involve a failure to mineralize the organic matrix elaborated by osteoblasts, and in the case of children by the chondroblasts of the epiphyseal plate. In children, there is a very rapid elaboration of organic matrix and an elongation of bone involving epiphyseal plate growth. It appears that the recruitment of the chondrocytes and osteoblasts is not vitamin D–dependent, and the elaboration of organic matrix is also not defective in vitamin D deficiency. However, the primary defect is the failure to deposit calcium and phosphorus in the form of hydroxyapatite on the collagen fibrils [16,17]. In the absence of this mineral component, the collagen fibrils are unable to carry out the structural role of the skeleton, and bending and twisting occur in the case of the young where there are large amounts of this uncalcified and hence soft and pliable matrix [1,15].

The major reason for failure to mineralize the bone matrix in vitamin D deficiency is an inadequate supply of calcium and phosphorus in the plasma [16,17]. Although the suggestion has been made that vitamin D plays an important role in the actual mineralization process, so far direct evidence is lacking, although clinical evidence is suggestive [18]. There have been reports that claim to prove that vitamin D is not required for the mineralization of organic matrix of the skeleton by direct action, but these experiments are inconclusive and require additional work [19].

The essence of vitamin D action, therefore, is the elevation of plasma calcium and phosphorus to supersaturating levels required for bone mineralization. To carry out this role, vitamin D is involved in several basic processes. The best known is that vitamin D stimulates an active intestinal calcium absorption mechanism [20]. This is, as far as is known today, a system that is responsive only to the vitamin D hormone. Phosphate is a normal accompanying anion, and in addition there is a phosphate-oriented active transport mechanism induced in the epithelium of the small intestine to cause an elevation of plasma phosphorus as well [21–23].

In addition to the intestinal site, vitamin D is active in permitting the mobilization of calcium from the bone fluid compartment to the plasma [24]. This process involves not only the vitamin D hormone but also the parathyroid hormone with the vitamin D hormone acting in a permissive role, inducing machinery that is then responsive to the parathyroid hormone [25]. Both hormones are then required to mobilize calcium from bone to support plasma levels. Finally, in the distal renal tubule, there appears to be an interaction between the vitamin D hormone and parathyroid hormone in the final renal conservation of calcium [26,27]. Calcium is reabsorbed to the extent of 99 percent in the total absence of vitamin D and the parathyroid hormone. The remaining 1 percent that is reabsorbed in the distal renal tubule is under control of these two humoral agents.

A diagrammatic illustration of these mechanisms is shown in Figure 4-3. By these mechanisms, plasma calcium and phosphorus are raised to levels that will (1) provide adequate amounts of calcium for the neuromuscular junction and for nerves and muscles to operate, and (2) provide sufficient amounts of calcium to support the mineralization of bone. In order to carry out these functions, vitamin D must be metabolically altered to produce a hormone, as discussed in the next section.

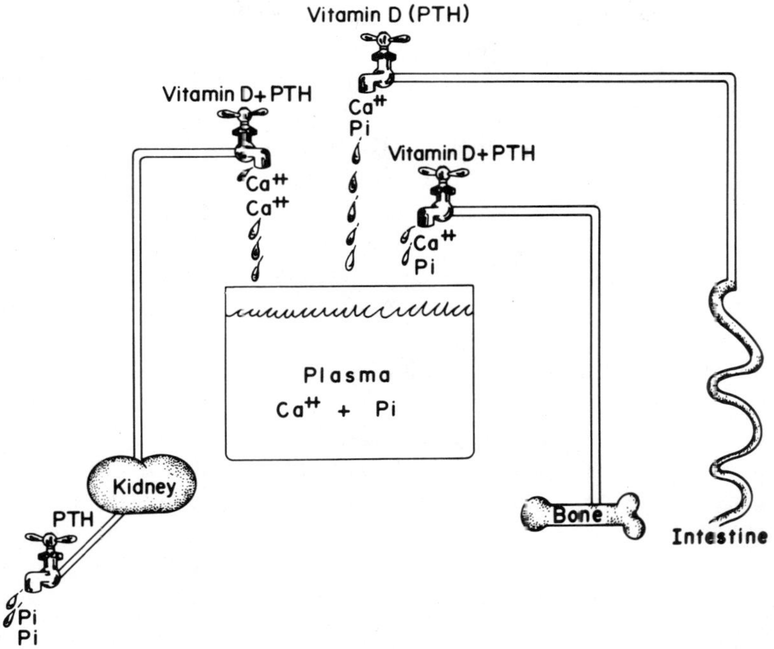

Figure 4-3. Sites of action of vitamin D. PTH is parathyroid hormone. Note that parathyroid hormone [(PTH)] written over the pump for the intestine is not directly involved in stimulating this transport phenomenon but instead is involved in the conversion of vitamin D to its active form, which then activates the intestine to transport calcium.

Metabolism of Vitamin D to Its Hormonal Form

Vitamin D accumulates specifically in the liver, in contrast to other forms of vitamin D, namely its metabolites [11,28]. In the endoplasmic reticulum or microsomes, vitamin D is converted to its major circulating form, 25-hydroxyvitamin D (25-OH-D), as illustrated in Figure 4-4. This reaction depends on a cytochrome P-450 enzyme that is not inducible by drugs such as phenobarbital or diphenylhydantoin (Dilantin) [29]. This major circulating form is not active directly but must be further metabolically altered. The second alteration takes place in the kidney [30] and, for all practical purposes, in the nonpregnant mammal exclusively so in that organ [31]. There, 25-OH-D is converted in the mitochondria to 1,25-hydroxyvitamin D_3 (1,25-$(OH)_2D_3$) by an NADPH, cytochrome P-450-dependent reaction [32]. 1,25-$(OH)_2D_3$, which is the product of this sequence, is then transferred to the target organs intestine, bone, and elsewhere in the kidney where it stimulates the transport reactions described in the previous section. The enzymatic machinery involved in the 1-hydroxylation of 25-OH-D is quite similar to the adrenal hormone-producing systems in the adrenal glands [32]. It is this enzyme that is regulated in true endocrine fashion.

The basis for concluding that 1,25-$(OH)_2D_3$ or a further metabolite is the hormonal form of vitamin D is the observation by Fraser and Kodicek that the kidney is virtually the exclusive site of synthesis of 1,25-$(OH)_2D_3$ in the nonpregnant mammal [30]. Thus, it has been shown that if kidneys are removed from vitamin D–deficient rats, their intestinal calcium transport or bone calcium mobilization systems do not respond to 25-OH-D given in physiologic doses, but they will respond to 1,25-$(OH)_2D_3$ in a fashion identical with the response seen in animals with intact kidneys [33–35]. These results illustrate that the kidney conversion of 25-OH-D to 1,25-$(OH)_2D_3$ is required for vitamin D to exert its activity. It is quite apparent that this does not exclude the possibility that 1,25-$(OH)_2D_3$ is further metabolized for function. This question has been examined carefully in two laboratories, and it has been shown that the lipid extracts of intestine and bone at the time they respond to radio-labeled vitamin D hormone contain in the lipid fraction only the vitamin D hormone [36,37]. Forty percent of the 1,25-$(OH)_2D_3$, however, is found in a water-soluble form that has been isolated and identified as a C_{23} carboxylic acid called calcitroic acid [38]. This compound is biologically inactive in comparison to the 1,25-$(OH)_2D_3$ that is ten times more active than the parent vitamin D substance [39]. Thus, it appears that 1,25-$(OH)_2D_3$ and not a further metabolite is the hormonal form of the vitamin. Calcitroic acid is a major biliary excretory product of the vitamin D hormone [40].

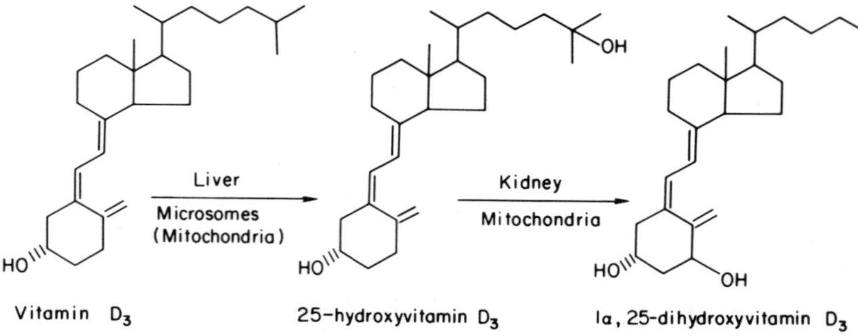

Figure 4-4. Metabolism of vitamin D required for function. Note that 1,25-$(OH)_2D_3$ for all practical purposes is made exclusively in the kidney and has its function in intestine, bone, and elsewhere in the kidney. In addition to the kidney as a site of 1α-hydroxylation, placenta has now been shown to produce the vitamin D hormone.

There have been reports that there are extrarenal sites of production of 1,25-$(OH)_2D_3$ [41–43]. Clearly, in pregnant mammals there is extrarenal production of 1,25-$(OH)_2D_3$ [41]. The site of this production is the placenta, and in fact, 25-OH-D-1α-hydroxylase has been clearly demonstrated in vitro in placental tissue [44]. However, there have been other reports claiming that bone cells and other organs are able to convert 25-OH-D to 1,25-$(OH)_2D_3$ [43,45]. Although this may have occurred in vitro in cultures of cells taken from those organs, or it may have occurred in some small degree in anephric patients on long-term hemodialysis [46] or in diseases such as sarcoidosis in which there is ectopic formation of 1,25-$(OH)_2D_3$ [47], this must not be misconstrued to mean that there is widespread production of 1,25-$(OH)_2D_3$. In fact, in normal anephric animals in the nonpregnant state there is little or no production of 1,25-$(OH)_2D_3$ as shown experimentally. Furthermore, target organs of anephric rats, such as bone, do not respond to 25-OH-D but do respond to 1,25-$(OH)_2D_3$ [33,34]. Obviously, if bone possessed the ability to carry out significant 1α-hydroxylation, the requirement for kidney 1α-hydroxylation would not have been shown. For all practical purposes, therefore, the site of production of the final vitamin D hormone is in the kidney and placenta.

Other Metabolism of Vitamin D_3

Vitamin D_3 is metabolized to a variety of other metabolic products, but all of them proceed through the major blood circulating form of vitamin D, namely 25-OH-D [48]. Figure 4-5 illustrates the major known in vivo metabolites of vitamin D [48]. This figure purposely excludes the reports of many other metabolites of vitamin D that have either been isolated or identified in animals given large amounts of vitamin D or that have been produced in vitro and have not been shown to occur in vivo. Clearly, a molecule such as the vitamin D structure having the unstable triene structure is easily isomerized, oxidized, and altered in in vitro circumstances in a way that perhaps does not occur in vivo.

In any case, the most important known additional pathways to vitamin D metabolism are (1) 26-hydroxylation to form the 25S,26-$(OH)_2D_3$, (2) 24R-hydroxylation to form 24R,25-$(OH)_2D_3$, and (3) 23S-hydroxylation, which forms an intermediate in the synthesis of 25-OH-D-26,23-lactone. The lactone and the 25,26-$(OH)_2D_3$ compounds are all much less biologically active than their precursor, 25-OH-D_3, and it is generally believed either that they are minor metabolites or that they have a role in the inactivation and excretion of the vitamin D molecule [48]. There has been considerable interest in findings that 24R,25-$(OH)_2D_3$ plays an important role in the mineralization of bone [49], in the suppression of parathyroid hormone secretion [50], or in

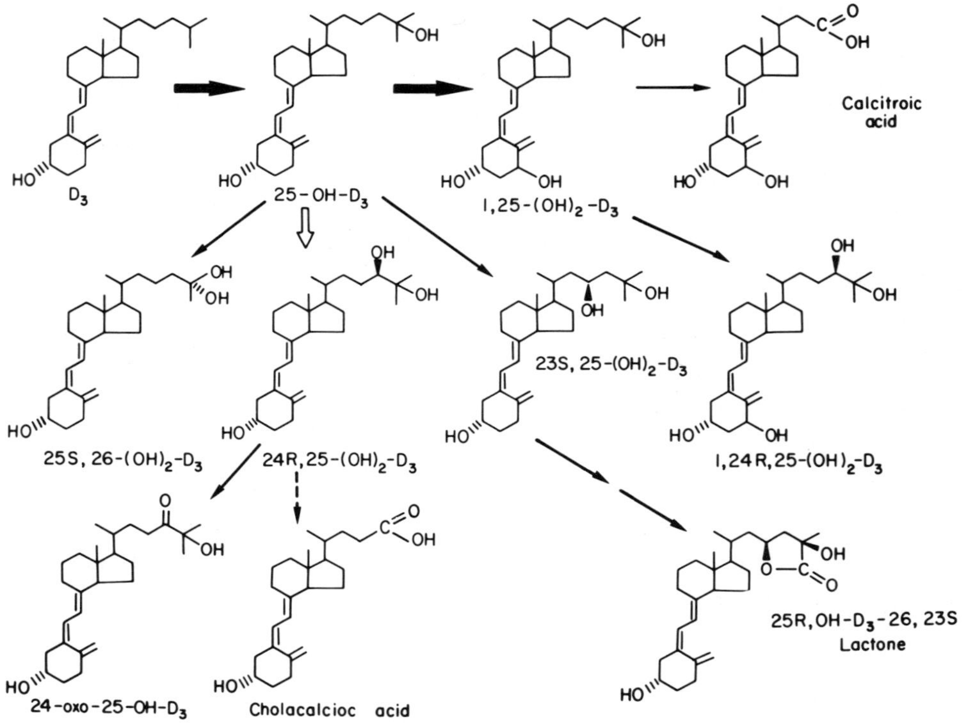

Figure 4-5. Overall metabolism of vitamin D illustrating the known in vivo pathways. The dark heavy arrows are the activation reactions; the clear arrow indicates major reactions of unknown physiologic significance. All other pathways are minor. The dotted pathway represents a reaction discovered only in vitro systems and not shown to occur in vivo.

embryonic development [51]. This compound has also received attention as a potential therapeutic agent in the treatment of bone disease. However, experiments in animals using 24,24-F_2-25-OH-D_3 or 1,25-$(OH)_2D_3$ delivered by osmotic minipump in a controlled fashion have shown that all of the biologic activities of vitamin D can be satisfied by compounds that cannot be 24-hydroxylated [48,52,53; unpublished results]. Thus, it is unlikely that 24R-hydroxylation plays any significant physiologic role in the expression of vitamin D action. Similar experiments have been carried out with 26,26,26, 27,27,27-F_6-25-OH-D_3, a compound that cannot be converted either to the lactone or the 25,26-$(OH)_2D_3$ compound [54]. Thus, it is apparent that at this point, the only activation steps for the vitamin D molecule are 25-hydroxylation and 1α-hydroxylation to produce the final vitamin D hormone, 1κ,25-$(OH)_2D_3$.

Mechanism of Action of 1,25-$(OH)_2D_3$

In the absence of evidence for other hormonal forms of vitamin D, this section will be devoted entirely to the concept that 1α,25-$(OH)_2D_3$ is the hormonal form of the vitamin in carrying out its well-known physiologic actions. It is now known both for the osteoblasts of bone and for the villus and crypt cells of the intestine that 1,25-$(OH)_2D_3$ accumulates in the nucleus of these cells prior to initiation of the biologic responses [55,56]. This can be shown by means of tritium-labeled 1,25-$(OH)_2D_3$ and freeze-thaw autoradiography, or by biochemical means. Nuclear localization of 1,25-$(OH)_2D_3$ in intestinal villus cells is illustrated in Figure 4-6. Thus, a nuclear-mediated mechanism of action of 1,25-$(OH)_2D_3$ can be expected. In agreement with this, a specific protein can be found in the target organs of 1,25-$(OH)_2D_3$ action that will bind specifically 1,25-$(OH)_2D_3$ with a K_D of about 5×10^{-11}M [57,58]. This macromolecule is highly specific for 1,25-$(OH)_2D_3$. It has been isolated in

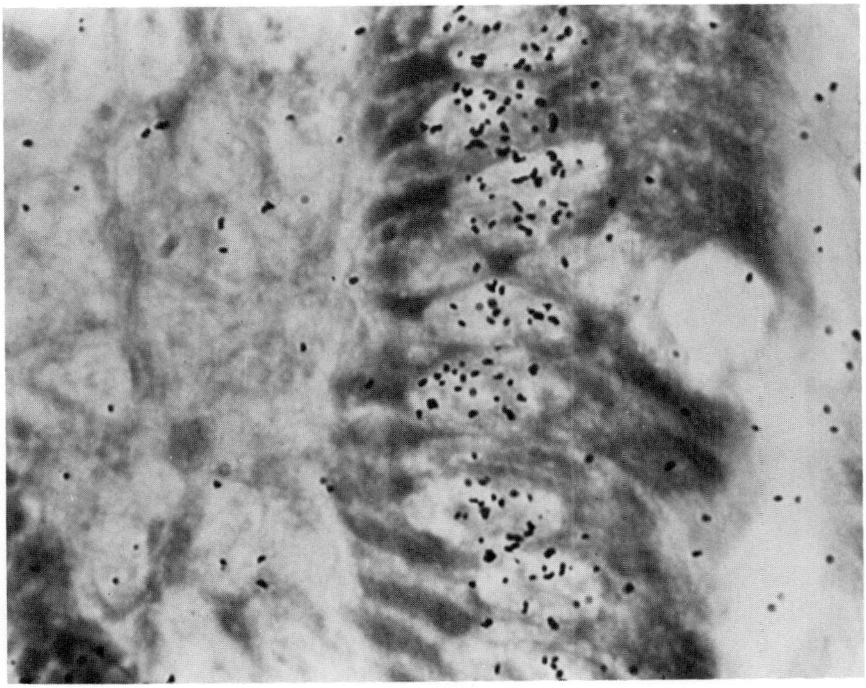

Figure 4-6. Localization of 1,25-$(OH)_2$[26,27-^{3}H]-D_3 in the intestinal villus cells. Note an absence of localization in the submucosa and goblet cells, but all localization in the villus cells is found in the nucleus.

pure form from the chick small intestine and shown to be a single polypeptide of 63,000 molecular weight possessing several sulfhydryl groups [59]. This receptor molecule has been used to determine the blood levels of 1,25-$(OH)_2D_3$ both in animals and in human patients [60]. This receptor-like molecule can be found in all known target organs [61], but in addition, it can now be found in a variety of other tissues and transformed cells such as cancer cell lines [61]. Nuclear localization of 1,25-$(OH)_2D_3$ and the existence of a receptor can be demonstrated, in addition to the small intestine, in the bone, kidney, skin, endocrine cells of the stomach, pituitary, parathyroid glands, and islet cells of the pancreas [61]. Some evidence for a role of the vitamin D hormone has been presented for skin [62], parathyroid glands [63], and the islet cells of the pancreas [64]. Thus, it is becoming apparent that the vitamin D hormone not only may play an important role in regulating calcium and phosphorus metabolism of the plasma but also may be involved in other heretofore unknown mechanisms in such important organs such as the islet cells of the pancreas.

With the existence of a receptor and nuclear localization, it might be expected that transcription of DNA and protein synthesis must be involved in the expression of vitamin D action in the target organs. This has been a controversial area, in which there have been claims that the vitamin D hormone acts directly on the brush border surface to alter lipid composition without nuclear interaction [65,66]. To support this theory, it has been shown that actinomycin D, an inhibitor of transcription, does not block the intestinal responses to 1,25-$(OH)_2D_3$ [67]. However, these experiments lack sufficient support, since only 30 percent of the messenger RNA synthesis of the small intestine is blocked under the circumstances where the action of 1,25-$(OH)_2D_3$ is not blocked. Larger amounts of actinomycin D result in death of the animal, and hence conclusions are not possible. In organ cultures, however, it can be shown that cycloheximide, actinomycin D, α-amanitin, and anisomycin all block the intestinal calcium transport response to 1,25-$(OH)_2D_3$ added in vitro [68]. Furthermore, in the case of cycloheximide, this inhibition is clearly reversible, illustrating that the cells did not fail to transport calcium because of intoxication but rather because of a specific inhibition. Thus, the best current evidence suggests that transcription and protein synthesis are involved in the expression of 1,25-$(OH)_2D_3$ action on the small intestine. Figure 4-7 illustrates the best model of the mechanism of action of the vitamin D hormone on the small intestinal villus cell. As is illustrated, its activity appears to mimic that proposed for other steroid hormones, namely association with a receptor, appearance together with the receptor in the nucleus, and transcription of specific genes that code for calcium and phosphorus transport proteins. The messenger RNA is then translated and the formed proteins appear at the brush border surface and perhaps the basal-lateral membrane, where they initiate transfer reactions resulting in transcellular cal-

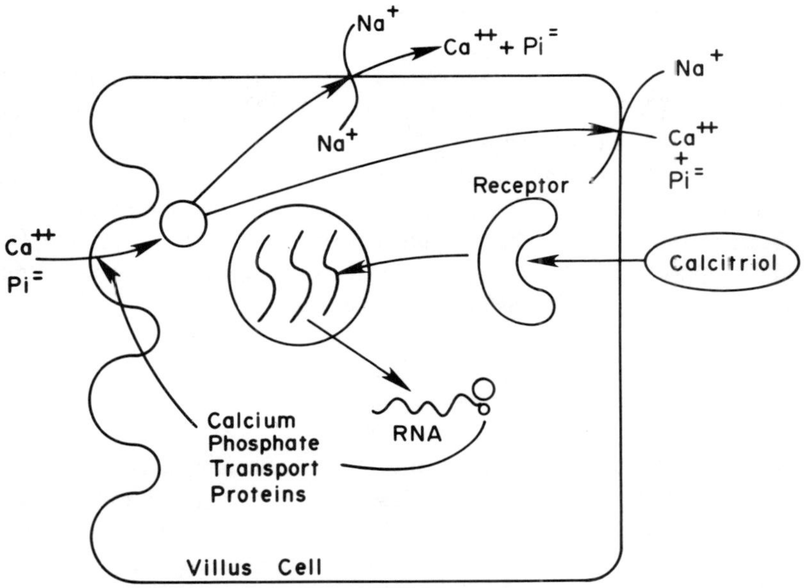

Figure 4-7. Expected molecular mechanism of action of 1,25-$(OH)_2D_3$ (calcitriol).

cium and phosphorus transport. Sodium is required at the basal-lateral membrane for expulsion of calcium, but beyond this, little is known concerning the molecular events of the transport. The only protein known to be formed in response to the vitamin D hormone is the calcium-binding protein discovered by Wasserman and his colleagues [69]. Exactly what role this protein has in calcium transport remains controversial and unclear.

There is strong evidence that the receptor mechanism is involved in the expression of 1,25-$(OH)_2D_3$ action. Clinical evidence is from a disease known as vitamin D–dependency rickets type II [70,71]. This disease is one in which the siblings present with severe rickets in the face of very high levels of blood 1,25-$(OH)_2D_3$. Furthermore, cells that are taken from these children and cultured show an absence of the receptor for the vitamin D hormone, whereas skin taken from subjects not having the disease shows clearly the presence of the receptor [72]. In addition, suckling rats do not possess the vitamin D–dependent intestinal calcium transport mechanism while they are consuming milk [73]. This correlates exactly with the absence of the 1,25-$(OH)_2D_3$ receptor [74]. At the time of weaning, the responsiveness to the vitamin D hormone makes its appearance in suckling rat pups, and correlates with the appearance of the receptor. These then constitute two lines of evidence supporting the idea of the mechanism proposed earlier for the action of vitamin D hormone in the target tissues.

Similar mechanisms can be expected in the bone, although very little has yet been elucidated except that the action of 1,25-$(OH)_2D_3$ in bone does require protein and RNA synthesis [75]. From the above discussion it is clear that the molecular mechanism of action of 1,25-$(OH)_2D_3$, as well as the fact that in nonpregnant animals 1,25-$(OH)_2D_3$ is essentially made exclusively in the kidney and sent to other organs where it expresses its activity, very strongly supports the idea that 1,25-$(OH)_2D_3$ is the hormonal form of vitamin D, with the kidney serving as an endocrine organ.

Control of Metabolism of Vitamin D

In normal mammals under conditions of hypocalcemia, production of the vitamin D hormone is markedly increased [76]. Under conditions of hypercalcemia, production of the vitamin D hormone is suppressed [76]. In an almost reciprocal fashion, 24,25-$(OH)_2D_3$ is not produced under conditions of hypocalcemia but is produced under conditions when 1α-hydroxylase is suppressed. Thus low blood calcium, and hence the need for calcium, stimulates production of the vitamin D hormone. This can be shown by direct measurements of the 25-OH-D-1α-hydroxylase in the kidney [77,78]. Parathyroidectomy eliminates response of the 1α-hydroxylase to the hypocalcemia [79]. This response can be restored by the injection of parathyroid hormone, and thus it is now quite apparent that the parathyroid glands primarily mediate the hypocalcemic stimulation of the vitamin D endocrine system in the kidney to produce the vitamin D hormone.

As illustrated in Figure 4-8 [80], the parathyroid glands monitor plasma calcium concentration and, in response to hypocalcemia, secrete parathyroid hormone. This 84-amino-acid peptide is then bound to the kidney and to bone. In the kidney, it blocks renal tubule reabsorption of phosphate, a function that is not dependent on the presence of vitamin D. On the other hand, in the same cell [81] it stimulates production of 1,25-$(OH)_2D_3$. In the distal renal tubule, the parathyroid hormone functions with existent 1,25-$(OH)_2D_3$ to stimulate renal reabsorption of calcium [26,27]. The stimulated 1α-hydroxylase produces 1,25-$(OH)_2D_3$ that travels to the small intestine, where it stimulates intestinal calcium and phosphate transport [20–23]. At the bone site, 1,25-$(OH)_2D_3$ permits parathyroid hormone to stimulate the transfer of calcium from the bone fluid compartment to the plasma [25]. These reactions then serve to elevate plasma calcium concentration, shutting off parathyroid hormone secretion which in turn shuts off production of the vitamin D hormone. In this manner, plasma calcium is kept in the normal range. It is clear, therefore, that the vitamin D endocrine system plays a central role in regulating the plasma calcium concentration.

In the thyroparathyroidectomized animal the 25-OH-D-1α-hydroxylase is suppressed, but if the animals are made hypophosphatemic by phosphate deprivation or glucose loading, then the 25-OH-D-1α-hydroxylase of the kidney is markedly enhanced, giving rise to high blood levels of 1,25-$(OH)_2D_3$ [82]. This in turn stimulates phosphate absorption in the small intestine, correcting the hypophosphatemia [21–23]. Therefore, 1,25-$(OH)_2D_3$ can also be regarded as a phosphate homeostatic hormone.

Of great importance is the essential role of the vitamin D endocrine system in protecting the skeleton from loss [83]. If there is a chronic need for calcium to calcify the skeleton or if there is a chronic loss of calcium, a normal

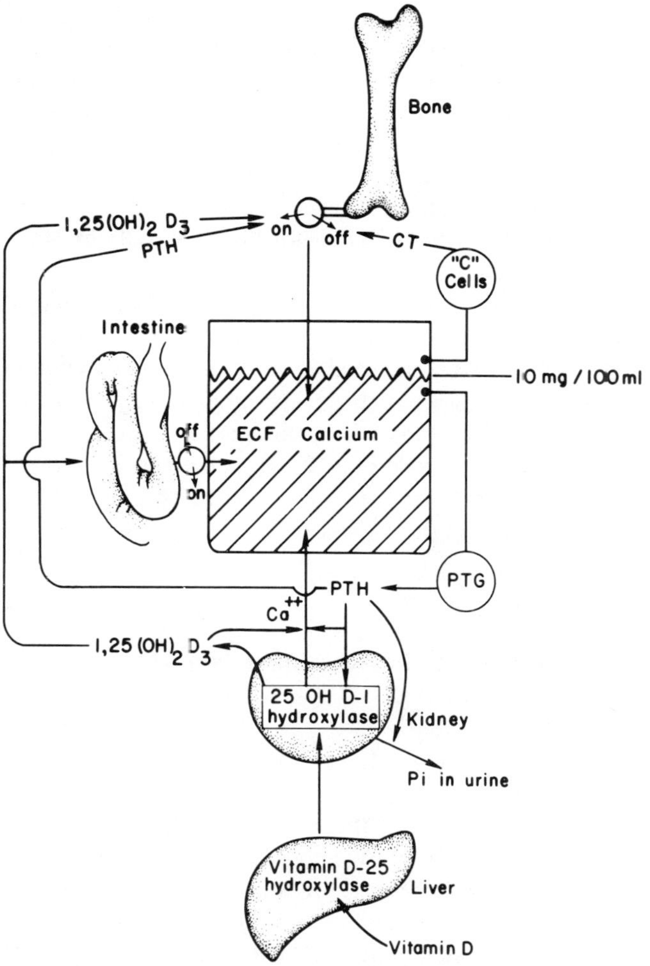

Figure 4-8. The calcium homeostatic mechanism involving the vitamin D endocrine system and the parathyroid gland.

sequence of events is stimulation of the parathyroid, which in turn stimulates 25-OH-D-1α-hydroxylase that produces 1,25-$(OH)_2D_3$. The 1,25-$(OH)_2D_3$ stimulates the only organ that can sequester calcium from the environment, namely the small intestine [20]. This phenomenon was originally ascribed to an unknown factor called the Nicolaysen endogenous factor [84]. If the efficiency of calcium absorption is not increased in response to the need for calcium, there will be an increasing reliance on skeletal calcium to meet the needs of soft tissue [83,84]. This situation, if it persists, will result in loss of bone mass, giving rise to osteopenia that might then result in symptomatic osteoporosis. Thus the vitamin D endocrine system is essential in calcium economy of the organism, and it is in this area that the most widespread of the bone diseases is believed to result, namely the osteoporoses.

In addition to these mechanisms whereby the vitamin D hormone production is stimulated by the need for calcium or phosphorus, increased production is required in conditions such as pregnancy and lactation and the production of eggs and egg shells in birds. Under these circumstances, the vitamin D endocrine system has been shown to react in an appropriate way to bring about increased production of the vitamin D hormone and hence increased mobilization of calcium to meet these demands [85–87]. In addition to these mechanisms, the vitamin D hormone itself stimulates 25-OH-D-24R-hydroxylase in the kidney and suppressed the 25-OH-D-1α-hydroxylase in the kidney [88]. The mechanism of this regulation is not understood, except it is believed to involve a nuclear process [89]. In addition to this process, other endocrine systems have been reported to interact with the vitamin D endocrine system in circumstances such as hypophysectomy, bringing about a reduced production of the vitamin D hormone that can be partially restored by the injection of growth hormone [90,91]. One can expect an increased number of findings on the interaction between the vitamin D endocrine system and other endocrines in the regulation of calcium and phosphorus metabolism.

Diseases Resulting from Disturbances in the Vitamin D Endocrine System

Hypoparathyroidism and Pseudohypoparathyroidism

Early in the course of discovery of the vitamin D endocrine system, it became apparent that the vitamin D hormone could be extremely useful in the treatment of hypoparathyroid diseases. In this disorder, it is clear that the calcium-sensing organ of the body has been lost either by surgery or by genetic or other causes [92]. Such patients develop hypocalcemia without consequent elevation of the plasma 1,25-$(OH)_2D_3$ levels [93]. This results in a hypocalcemic tetany easily diagnosed by the physician. Treatment of this disorder is best accomplished by administration of the vitamin D hormone that stimulates the small intestine, not requiring the presence of the parathyroid hormone. To ensure that the intestine can support plasma calcium concentration, large amounts of dietary calcium are also prescribed. Thus, treatment is best accomplished by the administration of approximately 1 g of oral calcium in the form of calcium carbonate or calcium gluconate and approximately 1 μg of 1,25-$(OH)_2D_3$ per day [94,95]. In some hypoparathyroid patients, large doses of 1,25-$(OH)_2D_3$ have been necessary [96]. The reason for this apparent resistance is unknown.

Pseudohypoparathyroidism is a disorder in which parathyroid secretion occurs normally in response to hypocalcemia but the target organs do not respond to the secreted parathyroid hormone. This results in low plasma 1,25-$(OH)_2D_3$ levels and a hypocalcemia [93]. This disorder is efficiently treated by the administration of oral calcium and the vitamin D hormone [94,95]. So successful has been the use of the vitamin D hormone for the treatment of hypoparathyroidism that it is clearly the method of choice. In fact, the prescription of large doses of ordinary vitamin D for the treatment of this disorder should be discontinued because of the great danger of intoxication of the patient. It is known that vitamin D is stored in the fat depots [97], and when hypercalcemia due to hypervitaminosis results, it is difficult to correct the condition. In fact, this situation often results in persistent hypercalcemia, nephrocalcinosis, and aorta calcification. Since the vitamin D hormone has a short lifetime, if hypercalcemia results from its use, within one day or two after withdrawal of 1,25-$(OH)_2D_3$, hypercalcemia will disappear [94].

Renal Osteodystrophy

Loss of kidney function brings about two basic losses in the regulation of calcium and phosphorus metabolism [98]. First, the kidney is the primary organ that regulates the phosphorus level in the plasma [99]. Upon loss of nephrons, there is an increased phosphate retention resulting in suppression of ionized calcium and increased parathyroid hormone secretion, which then diminishes phosphate reabsorption in the remaining nephrons [100]. Nevertheless, there is a persistent secondary hyperparathyroidism that results [100]. Another major difficulty in the disorder is loss of the organ responsible for secreting the vitamin D hormone, namely the kidney [30]. This results in failure to absorb calcium, failure to mobilize calcium adequately, a hypocalcemia, and an osteomalacia. The failure to absorb calcium also contributes to the secondary hyperparathyroidism, and although it has been claimed that the lack of vitamin D hormone is not the early cause of bone disease [101], this is not entirely clear since very early in the disease, the ratio of parathyroid hormone to vitamin D hormone in the plasma changes significantly [102]. It is at this stage that the source of calcium to support soft tissue needs shifts from the intestine to the bone. In any case, the use of the vitamin D hormone or its analogue, 1α-OH-D_3, has been very successful in managing the bone disease secondary to renal failure [48]. Doses of the order of 0.5 to 1 μg per day given in divided doses have been very useful in management of this disorder. However, 10 percent of the renal failure patients who present with an osteomalacia are resistant to treatment with the vitamin D hormone [48]. The reason for this remains unknown, although there has been recent success with parenteral administration of the vitamin D hormone to such patients. It has also been found that the use of large amounts of a vitamin D analogue such as 24,25-$(OH)_2D_3$ appears to diminish the hypercalcemic response to the vitamin D hormone [48]. Nevertheless, use of the vitamin D hormone has been successful in approximately 90 percent of cases in the treatment of this disorder.

Vitamin D–Resistant Rickets

The form of vitamin D–resistant rickets that involves a clear disorder in production of the vitamin D hormone is called vitamin D–dependency rickets type I [103]. It is an autosomal recessive condition in which the child presents with rickets with normal intakes of vitamin D and normal blood levels of 25-OH-D [103]. These patients present with low plasma levels of 1,25-$(OH)_2D_3$ [104], and their rickets is totally healed by the administration of physiologic amounts of exogenous 1,25-$(OH)_2D_3$ [103,105]. Although this disorder is likely to be a genetic defect in the gene expressing for 1α-hydroxylation, this has not been absolutely proved.

Another vitamin D–resistant condition related to vitamin D metabolism and function is vitamin D–dependency rickets type II, which is an autosomal recessive disorder in which children present with severe rickets, hypocalcemia, hypophosphatemia, and alopecia [70,71]. These patients, on examination, present with high blood levels of 1,25-$(OH)_2D_3$ in spite of the fact that they have large amounts of uncalcified osteoid. This disorder is clearly a target organ resistance to the vitamin D hormone, and it has recently been shown by Marx and his colleagues that cells obtained from such patients have no measureable receptor for 1,25-$(OH)_2D_3$, while cells obtained from normal subjects in the same way clearly possess the receptor [72]. Treatment of this disorder is by administration of large amounts of calcium, phosphorus, and the vitamin D hormone, with only limited success.

The most common of the vitamin D–resistant conditions is the X-linked hypophosphatemic vitamin D–resistant rickets [106]. There is no doubt that this disorder is one in which there is an enormous loss of phosphate in the urine due to a failure of renal reabsorption of phosphate [107]. This defect is not the result of a disorder in vitamin D metabolism, since there is no evidence to support the idea that a form of vitamin D has any influence on renal reabsorption of phosphorus [99]. However, these patients often present with low intestinal absorption of calcium, and if they are treated with inorganic phosphorus to increase their plasma phosphorus concentration and to correct their failure to mineralize bone, mineralization occurs in the epiphyseal plate but the patients develop a secondary hyperparathyroidism and a hypocalcemia [108]. It is now clear that these patients have low blood levels of 1,25-$(OH)_2D_3$, especially in the face of such low levels of blood inorganic phosphorus [104,109]. It seems that they have a primary defect in renal tubular reabsorption of phosphate and a secondary defect in the signal for stimulating 25-OH-D-1α-hydroxylase. These patients are best treated by frequent oral doses of phosphate on the order of 1.5 g per day, and then the administration of the vitamin D hormone on the order of 0.5 to 1 μg per day to correct for diminished calcium absorption and secondary hyperparathyroidism [108,110]. These patients then show not only well-mineralized bone following treatment, but also increased growth rate.

Osteoporosis

The most widespread of all the disorders suffered by man in the area of bone disease is osteoporosis. There are three general types: glucocorticoid-induced osteoporosis, involutional osteoporosis, and the postmenopausal type of osteoporosis. With the discovery of the vitamin D endocrine system has come a renewed interest in the possibility that these bone diseases might in part be the result of a disordered vitamin D metabolism. There is no doubt that the stimulation of intestinal calcium absorption under conditions where the subject requires calcium is an important mechanism for protecting against skeletal loss of calcium [83]. It is well known that if insufficient amounts of calcium are absorbed in the small intestine, calcium will be removed from bone to support soft tissue needs. Of particular importance, therefore, is the fact that there is a marked decrease in intestinal calcium absorption efficiency as a function of age [111–113]. This exactly correlates with a decreased blood level of 1,25-$(OH)_2D_3$. Administration of 1,25-$(OH)_2D_3$ to elderly patients stimulates intestinal calcium transport or absorption, illustrating that responsiveness is still present [111,113]. Involutional osteoporosis then could be in part a failure to absorb calcium and a failure to produce sufficient amounts of 1,25-$(OH)_2D_3$ to meet the calcium needs of the organism. This results in increased reliance on skeletal calcium stores, giving rise to thin bones, osteoporosis, and fractures. So far, neither the glucocorticoid-induced osteoporosis nor the involutional type have been treated with the vitamin D hormone.

Table 4-1
Plasma 1,25-$(OH)_2D_3$ Levels in Postmenopausal Osteoporotic Patients

Subject	*1,25-$(OH)_2D_3$*	*1,25-/25- × 10^3* [a]
Healthy controls (age 50-65; n = 20)	35.2 ± 2.3	2.48 ± 0.25
Osteoporotic patients (age 50-65; n = 25)	25.8 ± 1.4 [b]	1.56 ± 0.17 [c]

[a] 1,25- = 1,25-dihydroxyvitamin D_3; 25- = hydroxyvitamin D_3.
[b] Significantly different from control, $p < 0.005$.
[c] Significantly different from control, $p < 0.001$.

By far the largest group of osteoporotic subjects is postmenopausal women [114]. There is a 30-percent decrease in plasma levels of 1,25-$(OH)_2D_3$ in this group, as shown in Table 4-1. This correlates with a 30-percent decrease in intestinal calcium absorption. Furthermore, osteoporotic women when shifted to a low-calcium diet do not show an increased rate of intestinal calcium absorption, illustrating that the physiologic response to a need for calcium is not adequate in these patients [111]. Thus, at least in part, some of the disorder can come from defective production of 1,25-$(OH)_2D_3$ to meet calcium needs of the postmenopausal woman. However, it is likely that the primary insult resulting in the osteoporosis is an increased loss of bone upon withdrawal of estrogens and testosterone as a result of the postmenopausal state [115]. Calcium coming from the skeleton then suppresses parathyroid hormone secretion and probably suppresses production of 1,25-$(OH)_2D_3$. This in turn diminishes intestinal calcium absorption, providing increased dependence on bone calcium for soft tissue needs. It is, therefore, of some interest to determine whether intervention could be adequately achieved by the administration of exogenous vitamin D hormone. One trial has been completed at the Mayo Clinic, carried out in a double-blind fashion in which osteoporotic women were treated either with a placebo or with 0.5 μg per day of 1,25-$(OH)_2D_3$ [116]. At the end of six months, the treated group showed a marked improvement in calcium retention and balance, whereas the untreated group continued to lose 60 mg of calcium per day. At this time the untreated group was shifted to treatment, and after two years they were examined again. At the end of two years, both increased intestinal absorption and improved calcium balance persisted, although the latter was not as positive as it had been at the six-month period. Of great importance is the finding that there was an increase in histologically detectable trabecular bone volume and a diminished fracture rate (Table 4-2). Thus, use of the vitamin D hormone for the treatment of osteoporosis in the postmenopausal woman seems

Table 4–2
Postmenopausal Osteoporosis:
Treatment with 1,25-$(OH)_2D_3$ (0.5 μg/day)

Measures of Bone Metabolism	*Time After Initiation of Treatment*		
	Baseline	*6–8 Months*	*2 Years*
Calcium absorption (%)	7	27[a]	27[a]
Calcium balance (mg/day)	−59	2[b]	−27
Trabecular bone volume (%)	11.3	13.4	16.2[b]
Urinary hydroxyproline (mg/day)	26.3	21.1[b]	22.0[b]

[a] $p < 0.001$.
[b] $p < 0.01$.

indicated. This has led to several large-scale trials by the Hoffmann-LaRoche Company, which is currently seeking evidence regarding the efficacy and safety of the vitamin D hormone in treating this disorder.

Summary

The vitamin D endocrine system is of great importance in calcium homeostasis, phosphorus homeostasis, and calcium economy of the body. There are disorders of these systems, including hypoparathyroidism, pseudohypoparathyroidism, vitamin D–resistant rickets, renal osteodystrophy, and the osteoporoses. It is clear that the vitamin D endocrine system will provide a new understanding of these disorders and that the vitamin D hormone and its analogues will provide a new mode of treatment for at least some of these conditions.

References

1. Mellanby, E. An experimental investigation on rickets. *Lancet* 1:407–412, 1919.

2. McCollum, E.V., Simmonds, N., Becker, J.E., Shipley, P.G. Studies on experimental rickets: XXI. An experimental demonstration of the existence of a vitamin which promotes calcium deposition. *J. Biol. Chem.* 53:293–312, 1922.

3. Huldshinsky, K. Heilung von Rachitis durch Künstliche Höhensonne. *Dtsch. Med. Wochenschr.* 45:712–713, 1919.

4. Steenbock, H. The induction of growth promoting and calcifying properties in a ration by exposure to light. *Science* 60:224–225, 1924.

5. Askew, F.A., Bourdillon, R.B., Bruce, H.M., et al. The distillation of vitamin D. *Proc. Roy. Soc.* B107:76–90, 1931.

6. Windaus, A., Schenck, F., von Werder, F. Über das antirachitisch wirksame Bestrahlungs-produkt aus 7-dehydro-Cholesterin. *Hoppe-Seylers Z. Physiol. Chem.* 241:100–103, 1936.

7. Esvelt, R.P., Schnoes, H.K., DeLuca, H.F. Vitamin D_3 from rat skins irradiated *in vitro* with ultraviolet light. *Arch. Biochem. Biophys.* 188:282–286, 1978.

8. Holick, M.F., Richtand, N.M., McNeill, S.C., et al. Isolation and identification of previtamin D_3 from the skin of rats exposed to ultraviolet irradiation. *Biochemistry* 18:1003–1008, 1979.

9. Holick, M.F., Clark, M.B. The photobiogenesis and metabolism of vitamin D. *Fed. Proc.* 37:2567–2574, 1978.

10. Bouillon, R., Van Baelen, H., Rombauts, W., DeMoor, P. The purification and characterization of the human-serum binding protein for the 25-hydroxycholecalciferol (transcalciferin). Identity with group-specific component. *Eur. J. Biochem.* 66:285–291, 1976.

11. Ponchon, G., DeLuca, H.F. The role of the liver in the metabolism of vitamin D. *J. Clin. Invest.* 48:1273–1279, 1969.

12. Holick, M.F., MacLaughlin, J.A., Doppelt, S.H. Regulation of cutaneous previtamin D_3 photosynthesis in man: Skin pigment is not an essential regulator. *Science* 211:590–593, 1981.

13. Rasmussen, H., DeLuca, H., Arnaud, C., et al. The relationship between vitamin D and parathyroid hormone. *J. Clin. Invest.* 42:1940–1946, 1963.

14. Harrison, H.E., Harrison, H.C. The interaction of vitamin D and parathyroid hormone on calcium phosphorus and magnesium homeostasis in the rat. *Metabolism* 13:952–958, 1964.

15. Hess, A. The history of rickets. In Hess, A. (Ed.), *Rickets, Including Osteomalacia and Tetany*. Philadelphia: Lea and Febiger, 1929. Pp. 22–37.

16. Lamm, M., Neuman, W.F. On the role of vitamin D in calcification. *Arch. Pathol.* 66:204–209, 1958.

17. DeLuca, H.F. Mechanism of action and metabolic fate of vitamin D. *Vitam. Horm.* 25:315–367, 1967.

18. Eastwood, J.B., Harris, E., Stamp, T.C.B., De Wardener, H.E. Vitamin-D deficiency in the osteomalacia of chronic renal failure. *Lancet* 2:1322–1326, 1976.

19. Howard, G.A., Baylink, D.J. Matrix formation and osteoid maturation in vitamin D-deficient rats made normocalcemic by dietary means. *Min. Electrolyte Metab.* 3:44, 1980.

20. DeLuca, H.F. Vitamin D and calcium transport. In Scarpa, A.,

Carafoli, E. (Eds.), *Calcium Transport and Cell Function*, vol. 307. New York: New York Academy of Sciences, 1978. Pp. 356–376.

21. Chen, T.C., Castillo, L., Korycka-Dahl, M., DeLuca, H.F. Role of vitamin D metabolites in phosphate transport of rat intestine. *J. Nutr.* 104:1056–1060, 1974.

22. Harrison, H.E., Harrison, H.C. Intestinal transport of phosphate: Action of vitamin D, calcium, and potassium. *Am. J. Physiol.* 201:1007–1012, 1961.

23. Wasserman, R.H., Taylor, A.N. Intestinal absorption of phosphate in the chick: Effect of vitamin D_3 and other parameters. *J. Nutr.* 103:586–599, 1973.

24. Carlsson, A. Tracer experiments on the effect of vitamin D on the skeletal metabolism of calcium and phosphorus. *Acta Physiol. Scand.* 26:212–220, 1952.

25. Garabedian, M., Tanaka, Y., Holick, M.F., DeLuca, H.F. Response of intestinal calcium transport and bone calcium mobilization to 1,25-dihydroxyvitamin D_3 in thyroparathyroidectomized rats. *Endocrinology* 94:1022–1027, 1974.

26. Kleeman, C.R., Bernstein, D., Rockney, R., et al. Studies on the renal clearance of diffusible calcium and the role of the parathyroid glands in its regulation. In Greep, R.O., Talmage, R.V. (Eds.), *The Parathyroids.* Springfield, Ill.: Charles C Thomas, 1961. Pp. 353–387.

27. Sutton, R.A.L., Dirks, J.H. Renal handling of calcium. *Fed. Proc.* 37:2112–2119, 1978.

28. Bhattacharyya, M.H., DeLuca, H.F. The regulation of rat liver calciferol-25-hydroxylase. *J. Biol. Chem.* 248:2969–2973, 1973.

29. Madhok, T.C., DeLuca, H.F. Characteristics of the rat liver microsomal enzyme system converting cholecalciferol into 25-hydroxycholecalciferol. Evidence for the participation of cytochrome P-450. *Biochem. J.* 184:491–499, 1979.

30. Fraser, D.R., Kodicek, E. Unique biosynthesis by kidney of a biologically active vitamin D metabolite. *Nature* 228:764–766, 1970.

31. Gray, R., Boyle, I., DeLuca, H.F. Vitamin D metabolism: The role of kidney tissue. *Science* 172:1232–1234, 1971.

32. Ghazarian, J.G., Jefcoate, C.R., Knutson, J.C., et al. Mitochondrial cytochrome P_{450}: A component of chick kidney 25-hydroxycholecalciferol-1α-hydroxylase. *J. Biol. Chem.* 249:3026–3033, 1974.

33. Boyle, I.T., Miravet, L., Gray, R.W., et al. The response of intestinal calcium transport to 25-hydroxy and 1,25-dihydroxy vitamin D in nephrectomized rats. *Endocrinology* 90:605–608, 1972.

34. Wong, R.G., Norman, A.W., Reddy, C.R., Coburn, J.W. Biologic

effects of 1,25-dihydroxycholecalciferol (a highly active vitamin D metabolite) in acutely uremic rats. *J. Clin. Invest.* 51:1287–1291, 1972.

35. Holick, M.F., Garabedian, M., DeLuca, H.F. 1,25-Dihydroxycholecalciferol: A metabolite of vitamin D_3 active on bone in anephric rats. *Science* 176:1146–1147, 1972.

36. Frolik, C.A., DeLuca, H.F. 1,25-Dihydroxycholecalciferol: The metabolite of vitamin D responsible for increased intestinal calcium transport. *Arch. Biochem. Biophys.* 147:143–147, 1971.

37. Tsai, H.C., Wong, R.G., Norman, A.W. Studies on calciferol metabolism: IV. Subcellular localization of 1,25-dihydroxy-vitamin D_3 in intestinal mucosa and correlation with increased calcium transport. *J. Biol. Chem.* 247:5511–5519, 1972.

38. Esvelt, R.P., Schnoes, H.K., DeLuca, H.F. Isolation and characterization of 1α-hydroxy-tetranorvitamin D-23-carboxylic acid: A major metabolite of 1,25-dihydroxyvitamin D_3. *Biochemistry* 18:3977–3983, 1979.

39. Esvelt, R.P., DeLuca, H.F. Calcitroic acid: Biological activity and tissue distribution studies. *Arch. Biochem. Biophys.* 206:403–413, 1981.

40. Onisko, B.L., Esvelt, R.P., Schnoes, H.K., DeLuca, H.F. Metabolites of 1α,25-dihydroxyvitamin D_3 in rat bile. *Biochemistry* 19:4124–4130, 1980.

41. Gray, T.K., Lester, G.E., Lorenc, R.S. Evidence for extra-renal 1α-hydroxylation of 25-hydroxyvitamin D_3 in pregnancy. *Science* 204:1311–1313, 1979.

42. Weisman, R., Vargas, A., Duckett, G., et al. Synthesis of 1,25-dihydroxyvitamin D in the nephrectomized pregnant rat. *Endocrinology* 103:1992–1998, 1978.

43. Howard, G.A., Turner, R.T., Sherrard, D.J., Baylink, D.J. Human bone cells in culture metabolize 25-hydroxyvitamin D_3 to 1,25-dihydroxyvitamin D_3 and 24,25-dihydroxyvitamin D_3. *J. Biol. Chem.* 256:7738–7740, 1981.

44. Tanaka, Y., Halloran, B., Schnoes, H.K., DeLuca, H.F. In vitro production of 1,25-dihydroxyvitamin D_3 by rat placental tissue. *Proc. Natl. Acad. Sci. U.S.A.* 76:5033–5035, 1979.

45. Turner, R.T., Puzas, J.E., Forte, M.D., et al. In vitro synthesis of 1α,25-dihydroxycholecalciferol and 24,25-dihydroxycholecalciferol by isolated calvarial cells. *Proc. Natl. Acad. Sci. U.S.A.* 77:5720–5724, 1980.

46. Lambert, P.W., Stern, P., Avioli, R.C., et al. Evidence for extrarenal production of 1,25-dihydroxyvitamin D_3 in man. *J. Clin. Invest.* 69:722–725, 1982.

47. Barbour, G.L., Coburn, J.W., Slatopolsky, E., et al. Hypercalcemia in an anephric patient with sarcoidosis: Evidence for extrarenal generation of 1,25-dihydroxyvitamin D. *N. Engl. J. Med.* 305:440–443, 1981.

48. DeLuca, H.F. Metabolism and mechanism of action of vitamin D—

1982. In Peck, W.A. (Ed.), *Annual Advances in Bone and Mineral Research*, vol. 1. Amsterdam: Excerpta Medica, 1982.

49. Ornoy, A., Goodwin, D., Hoff, D., Edelstein S. 24,25-Dihydroxyvitamin D is a metabolite of vitamin D essential for bone formation. *Nature* 276:517–519, 1978.

50. Henry, H.L., Taylor, A.N., Norman, A.W. Response of chick parathyroid glands to the vitamin D metabolites 1,25-dihydroxyvitamin D_3 and 24,25-dihyroxyvitamin D_3. *J. Nutr.* 107:1918–1926, 1977.

51. Henry, H.L., Norman, A.W. Vitamin D: Two dihydroxylated metabolites are required for normal chicken egg hatchability. *Science* 201:835–837, 1978.

52. Tanaka, Y., DeLuca, H.F., Kobayashi, Y., et al. Biological activity of 24,24-difluoro-25-hydroxyvitamin D_3. Effect of blocking of 24-hydroxylation on the functions of vitamin D. *J. Biol. Chem.* 254:7163–7167, 1979.

53. Miller, S.C., Halloran, B.P. DeLuca, H.F., et al. Studies on the role fo 24-hydroxylation of vitamin D in the mineralization of cartilage and bone of vitamin D–deficient rats. *Calcif. Tissue Int.* 33:489–497, 1981.

54. Tanaka, Y., Pahuja, D.N., Wichmann, J.K., et al. 25-Hydroxy-26,26,26,27,27,27-hexafluorovitamin D_3: Biological activity in the rat. *Arch. Biochem. Biophys.* 218:134–141, 1982.

55. Stumpf, W.E., Sar, M., Reid, F.A., et al. Target cells for 1,25-dihydroxyvitamin D_3 in intestinal tract, stomach, kidney, skin, pituitary and parathyroid. *Science* 206:1188–1190, 1979.

56. Stumpf, W.E., Sar, M., DeLuca, H.F. Sites of action of 1,25 $(OH)_2$ vitamin D_3 identified by thaw-mount autoradiography. In Cohn, D.V., Talmage, R.V., Matthews, J.L. (Eds.), *Hormonal Control of Calcium Metabolism*. Amsterdam: Excerpta Medica, 1981. Pp. 222–229.

57. Kream, B.E., Jose, M.J.L., DeLuca, H.F. The chick intestinal cytosol binding protein for 1,25-dihydroxyvitamin D_3: A study of analog binding. *Arch. Biochem. Biophys.* 179:462–468, 1977.

58. Mellon, W.S., DeLuca, H.F. An equilibrium and kinetic study of 1,25-dihydroxyvitamin D_3 binding to chicken intestinal cytosol employing high specific activity 1,25-dihydroxy [^{3}H-26,27] vitamin D_3. *Arch. Biochem. Biophys.* 197:90–95, 1979.

59. Simpson, R.U., DeLuca, H.F. Purification of chicken intestinal receptor for 1α,25-dihydroxyvitamin D_3 to apparent homogeneity. *Proc. Natl. Acad. Sci. U.S.A.* 79:16–20, 1982.

60. Eisman, J.A., Hamstra, A.J., Kream, B.E., DeLuca, H.F. A sensitive, precise, and convenient method for determination of 1,25-dihydroxyvitamin D in human plasma. *Arch. Biochem. Biophys.* 176:235–243, 1976.

61. Franceschi, R.T., Simpson, R.U., DeLuca, H.F. Binding proteins for vitamin D metabolites: Serum carriers and intracellular receptors. *Arch. Biochem. Biophys.* 210:1–13, 1981.

62. Esvelt, R.P., DeLuca, H.F., Wichmann, J.K., et al. 1,25-Dihydroxyvitamin D_3 stimulated increase of 7,8-didehydrocholesterol levels in rat skin. *Biochemistry* 19:6158–6161, 1980.

63. Chertow, B.S., Baylink, D.J., Wergedal, J.E., et al. Decrease in serum immunoreactive parathyroid hormone in rats and in parathyroid hormone secretion in vitro by 1,25-dihydroxycholecalciferol. *J. Clin. Invest.* 56:668–678, 1975.

64. Norman, A.W., Frankel, B.J., Heldt, A.M., Grodsky, G.M. Vitamin D deficiency inhibits pancreatic secretion of insulin. *Science* 209:823–825, 1980.

65. Max, E.E., Goodman, D.B.P., Rasmussen H. Purification and characterization of chick intestine brush border membrane. Effects of 1α-(OH)-vitamin D_3 treatment. *Biochim. Biophys. Acta* 511:224–239, 1978.

66. Goodman, D.B.P., Haussler, M.R., Rasmussen H. Vitamin D_3 induced alteration of microvillar membrane lipid composition. *Biochem. Biophys. Res. Commun.* 46:80–86, 1972.

67. Bikle, D.D., Zolock, D.T., Morrissey, R.L., Herman, R.H. Independence of 1,25-dihydroxyvitamin D_3-mediated calcium transport from de novo RNA and protein synthesis. *J. Biol. Chem.* 253:484–488, 1978.

68. DeLuca, H.F., Franceschi, R.T., Halloran B.P., Massaro, E.R. Molecular events involved in the 1,25-dihydroxyvitamin D_3 stimulation of intestinal calcium transport. *Fed. Proc.* 41:66–71, 1982.

69. Wasserman, R.H., Corradino, R.A. Vitamin D, calcium, and protein synthesis. *Vitam. Horm.* 31:43–103, 1973.

70. Bell, N.H., Hamstra, A.J., DeLuca, H.F. Vitamin D-dependent rickets type II: Resistance of target organs to 1,25-dihydroxyvitamin D. *N. Engl. J. Med.* 298:996–999, 1978.

71. Rosen, J.F., Fleischman, A.R., Finberg, L., et al. Rickets with alopecia: An inborn error of vitamin D metabolism. *J. Pediatr.* 94:729–735, 1979.

72. Eil, E., Liberman, U.A., Rosen, J.F., Marx, S.J. A cellular defect in hereditary vitamin-D-dependent rickets type II: Defective nuclear uptake of 1,25-dihydroxyvitamin D in cultured skin fibroblasts. *N. Engl. J. Med.* 304:1588–1591, 1981.

73. Halloran, B.P., DeLuca, H.F. Calcium transport in the small intestine during early development: The role of vitamin D. *Am. J. Physiol.* 239:G473–G479, 1980.

74. Halloran, B.P., DeLuca, H.F. Appearance of the intestinal cytosolic receptor for 1,25-dihydroxyvitamin D_3 during neonatal development in the rat. *J. Biol. Chem.* 256:7338–7342, 1981.

75. Tanaka, Y., DeLuca, H.F. Bone mineral mobilization activity of 1,25-dihydroxycholecalciferol, a metabolite of vitamin D. *Arch. Biochem. Biophys.* 146:574–578, 1971.

76. Boyle, I.T., Gray, R.W., DeLuca, H.F. Regulation by calcium of *in vivo* synthesis of 1,25-dihydroxycholecalciferol and 21,25-dihydroxycholecalciferol. *Proc. Natl. Acad. Sci. U.S.A.* 68:2131–2134, 1971.

77. Omdahl, J.L., Gray, R.W., Boyle, I.T., et al. Regulation of metabolism of 25-hydroxycholecalciferol by kidney tissue in vitro by dietary calcium. *Nature* (*New Biol.*) 237:63–64, 1972.

78. Tanaka, Y., DeLuca, H.F. Measurement of mammalian 25-hydroxyvitamin D_3 24R- and 1α-hydroxylase. *Proc. Natl. Acad. Sci. U.S.A.* 78:196–199, 1981.

79. Garabedian, M., Holick, M.F., DeLuca, H.F., Boyle, I.T. Control of 25-hydroxycholecalciferol metabolism by the parathyroid glands. *Proc. Natl. Acad. Sci. U.S.A.* 69:1673–1676, 1972.

80. DeLuca, H.F. Vitamin D: The vitamin and the hormone. *Fed. Proc.* 33:2211–2219, 1974.

81. Brunette, M.G., Chan, M., Ferriere, C., Roberts, K.D. Site of 1,25-dihydroxyvitamin D_3 synthesis in the kidney. *Nature* 276:287–289, 1978.

82. Tanaka, Y., DeLuca, H.F. The control of 25-hydroxyvitamin D metabolism by inorganic phosphorus. *Arch. Biochem. Biophys.* 154:566–574, 1973.

83. DeLuca, H.F. Calcium metabolism. *Acta Orthop. Scand.* 46:286–314, 1975.

84. Boyle, I.T., Gray, R.W., Omdahl, J.L., DeLuca, H.F. Calcium control of the in vivo biosynthesis of 1,25-dihydroxyvitamin D_3: Nicolaysen's endogenous factor. In Taylor, S. (Ed.), *Endocrinology 1971.* London: Heinemann, 1972. Pp. 468–476.

85. Halloran, B.P., Barthell, E.N., DeLuca, H.F. Vitamin D metabolism during pregnancy and lactation in the rat. *Proc. Natl. Acad. Sci. U.S.A.* 76:5549–5553, 1979.

86. Boass, A., Toverud, S.U., McCain, T.A., et al. Elevated serum levels of 1α,25-dihydroxycholecalciferol in lactating rats. *Nature* 267:630–631, 1977.

87. Castillo, L., Tanaka, Y., Wineland, M.J., et al. Production of 1,25-dihydroxyvitamin D_3 and formation of medullary bone in the egg-laying hen. *Endocrinology* 104:1598–1601, 1979.

88. Tanaka, Y., Lorenc, R.S., DeLuca, H.F. The role of 1,25-dihydroxyvitamin D_3 and parathyroid hormone in the regulation of chick renal 25-hydroxyvitamin D_3-24-hydroxylase. *Arch. Biochem. Biophys.* 171:521–526, 1975.

89. Larkins, R.G., MacAuley, S.J. MacIntyre, I. Feedback control of vitamin D metabolism by nuclear action of 1,25-dihydroxyvitamin D_3 on the kidney. *Nature* 252:412–414, 1974.

90. Pahuja, D.N., DeLuca, H.F. Role of the hypophysis in the regulation of vitamin D metabolism. *Mol. Cell. Endocrinol.* 23:345–350, 1981.

91. Spanos, E., Barrett, D., MacIntyre, I., et al. Effect of growth hormone on vitamin D metabolism. *Nature* 273:246–247, 1978.

92. Avioli, L.V. The therapeutic approach to hypoparathyroidism. *Am. J. Med.* 57:34–42, 1974.

93. Haussler, M.R. Vitamin D: Metabolism, drug interactions and therapeutic applications in humans. In Hathcock, J.N., Coon, J. (Eds.), *Nutrition and Drug Interrelations.* New York: Academic Press, 1978. Pp. 717–750.

94. Kooh, S.W., Fraser, D., DeLuca H.F., et al. Treatment of hypoparathyroidism and pseudohypoparathyroidism with metabolites of vitamin D: Evidence for impaired conversion of 25-hydroxyvitamin D to 1α,25-dihydroxyvitamin D. *N. Engl. J. Med.* 293:840–844, 1975.

95. Neer, R.M., Holick, M.F., DeLuca, H.F., Potts, J.T., Jr. Effects of 1α-hydroxyvitamin D_3 and 1,25-dihydroxyvitamin D_3 on calcium and phosphorus metabolism in hypoparathyroidism. *Metabolism* 24:1403–1413, 1975.

96. Chesney, R.W., Horowitz, S.D., Kream, B.E., et al. Failure of conventional doses of 1α,25-dihydroxycholecalciferol to correct hypocalcemia in a girl with idiopathic hypoparathyroidism. *N. Engl. J. Med.* 297:1272–1275, 1977.

97. Rosenstreich, S.J., Rich, C., Volwiler, W. Deposition in and release of vitamin D_3 from body fat: Evidence for a storage site in the rat. *J. Clin. Invest.* 50:679–687, 1971.

98. DeLuca, H.F., Avioli, L.V. Renal osteodystrophy. In Black, D., Jones, N.F. (Eds.), *Renal Disease.* London: Blackwell Scientific, 1979. Pp. 766–803.

99. Bonjour, J.P., Preston, C., Fleisch, H. Effect of 1,25-dihydroxyvitamin-D_3 on renal handling of P_i in thyroparathyroidectomized rats. *J. Clin. Invest.* 60:1419–1428, 1977.

100. Slatopolsky, E., Rutherford, W.E., Hoffsten, P.E., et al. Nonsuppressible secondary hyperparathyroidism in chronic progressive renal disease. *Kidney Int.* 1:38–46, 1972.

101. Slatopolsky, E., Rutherford, W.E., Hruska, K., et al. How important is phosphate in the pathogenesis of renal osteodystrophy? *Arch. Intern. Med.* 138:848–852, 1978.

102. DeLuca, H.F. The biochemical basis of renal osteodystrophy and post-menopausal osteoporosis: A view from the vitamin D system. *Curr. Med. Res. Opin.* 7:279–293, 1981.

103. Fraser, D., Kooh, S.W., Kind, H.P., et al. Pathogenesis of hereditary vitamin D dependent rickets: An inborn error of vitamin D metabolism involving defective conversion of 25-hydroxyvitamin D to 1α,25-dihydroxyvitamin D. *N. Engl. J. Med.* 289:817–822, 1973.

104. Scriver, C.R., Reade, T.M., DeLuca, H.F., Hamstra, A.J. Serum 1,25-$(OH)_2D$ levels in normal subjects and in patients with hereditary rickets or bone disease. *N. Engl. J. Med.* 299:976–979, 1978.

105. Balsan, S.M., Garabedian, M., Sorgniard, R., et al. 1,25-Dihydroxyvitamin D_3 and 1α-hydroxyvitamin D_3 in children: Biologic and therapeutic effects in nutritional rickets and different types of vitamin D resistance. *Pediatr. Res.* 9:586–593, 1975.

106. Williams, T.F., Winter, R.W., Burnett, C.H. Familial (hereditary) vitamin D–resistant rickets with hypophosphatemia. In Stanbury, J.B., Wyngaarden, J.B., Fredrickson, D.S. (Eds.), *The Metabolic Basis of Inherited Disease*, 2nd ed. New York: McGraw-Hill, 1966. Pp. 1179–1204.

107. Glorieux, F., Scriver, C.R. Loss of a parathyroid-sensitive component of phosphate transport in X-linked hypophosphatemia. *Science* 175:997–1000, 1972.

108. Glorieux, F.H., Marie, P.J., Pettifor, J.M., Delvin, E.E. Bone response to phosphate salts, ergocalciferol, and calcitriol in hypophosphatemic vitamin D–resistant rickets. *N. Engl. J. Med.* 303:1023–1031, 1980.

109. Chesney, R.W., Mazess, R.B., Rose, P., et al. Supranormal 25-hydroxyvitamin D and subnormal 1,25-dihydroxyvitamin D: Their role in X-linked hypophosphatemic rickets. *Am. J. Dis. Child.* 134:140–143, 1980.

110. Chesney, R.W., Mazess, R.B., Rose, P., et al. Long-term influence of calcitriol (1,25$(OH)_2$-Vitamin D) and supplemental phosphate in X-linked hypophosphatemic rickets. *Pediatrics*. In press.

111. Gallagher, J.C., Riggs, B.L., Eisman, J., et al. Intestinal calcium absorption and serum vitamin D metabolites in normal subjects and osteoporotic patients. Effects of age and dietary calcium. *J. Clin. Invest.* 64:729–736, 1979.

112. Bullamore, J.R., Gallagher, J.C., Wilkinson, R., Nordin, B.E.C. Effects of age on calcium absorption. *Lancet* 2:535–537, 1970.

113. Horst, R.L., DeLuca, H.F., Jorgensen, N.A. The effect of age on calcium absorption and accumulation of 1,25-dihydroxyvitamin D_3 in intestinal mucosa of rats. *Metab. Bone Dis. Rel. Res.* 1:29–33, 1978.

114. Crilly, R., Horsman, A., Marshall, D.H., Nordin, B.E.C. Prevalence, pathogenesis and treatment of postmenopausal osteoporosis. *Aust. N.Z. J. Med.* 9:24–30, 1979.

115. Gallagher, J.C., Riggs, B.L., Eisman, J., et al. Impaired intestinal calcium absorption in postmenopausal osteoporosis: Possible role of vitamin D metabolites and PTH. *Clin. Res.* 24:360A, 1976.

116. Gallagher, J.C., Jerpbak, C.M., Jee, W.S.S., et al. 1,25-Dihydroxyvitamin D_3: Short- and long-term effects on bone and calcium metabolism in patients with postmenopausal osteoporosis. *Proc. Natl. Acad. Sci. U.S.A.* 79:3325–3329, 1982.

5 Drugs and Nutrients

Daphne A. Roe, M.D.

Our forebears in physiologic chemistry provided us with clear definitions of nutrients and drugs. It was accepted that nutrients were substances that were essential to the growth and maintenance of living systems and that were involved in biosynthetic processes; in contrast, drugs were foreign to the body and not required for its physiologic economy. Before embarking on a discussion of drug-nutrient interactions, it is pertinent to remark that today we recognize that micronutrients or macronutrients, when given in pharmacologic doses, can behave as drugs, not only in terms of their absorption and disposition but also with respect to toxicity. Furthermore, we have caloric sources that have pharmacologic effects. On the other hand, synthetic retinoids, generally considered as drugs, are close relatives of vitamin A and therefore have characteristics akin to nutrients.

In this book, however, which focuses on nutrition in the young and the elderly, it is academic to focus on niceties of distinction between nutrients and drugs. Rather, it is important to describe those interactions of drugs and nutrients that have clinical importance either because they impose a risk of loss of drug efficacy or drug toxicity, or because they lead to drug-induced nutritional deficiencies. The discussion in this chapter will draw on examples of drug-nutrient interactions that are of particular importance in the very young and the very old.

Effects of Food and Nutrients on Drug Absorption

Reduction in Drug Absorption with Food

It is known that several drugs from major drug groups are less well absorbed when given with food. Included are a number of antibiotics such as penicillins, ampicillin (but not the ampicillin ester), pivampicillin [1–3], and the tetracyclines [4]. Isoniazid, extensively used as a tuberculostatic agent, is also less well absorbed after food than in the fasting state [5]. Rifampin, which is now used both in the treatment of tuberculosis and in the treatment of leprosy, is also less available when given with food [6].

Melander has suggested that with some of these drugs, decreased bioavailability associated with food intake can be explained by the reduced gastric acidity in the fed state [7]. A higher pH can slow the dissolution of drug particles. Concomitant intake of antacids with these drugs also reduces bioavailability, presumably for the same reason [8,9].

Decreased absorption of tetracycline occurs when foods containing calcium, magnesium, iron, or zinc are taken within two hours of the time of intake of the drug. In this case it has been shown that the reason for impaired drug absorption is that mineral chelates are formed which reduce drug solubility and uptake [4]. Bone meal, now being taken as a calcium source, has the same effect on tetracycline absorption.

The bioavailability of L-dopa and methyldopa may be reduced when these drugs are taken with protein foods or protein hydrolysates in liquid formula diets. The reason is that these drugs are both amino acids, and when dietary amino acids are present in the intestine at the same time, absorption of the drug and dietary amino acids are competitive [1].

Enhancement of Drug Absorption with Food

There are, on the other hand, several groups of drugs that are better absorbed when taken with food. These drugs include dicumarol, hydrochlorothiazide, nitrofurantoin, hydralazine, the beta blockers propranolol and metoprolol, certain preparations of phenytoin (diphenylhydantoin), and griseofulvin. Mechanisms underlying the promotional effect of food on the bioavailability of these drugs vary. In certain of these drugs, such as hydrochlorothiazide, the promotional effect of food on absorption can be simulated by the administration of anticholinergic drugs, which slow gastric emptying time. It is therefore proposed in this case that food increases drug absorption because gastric emptying time is delayed, which would allow more time for dissolution of the drug before it passes into the intestine where most of the drug is absorbed [10–12]. In this context, it is of interest that absorption of pharmacologic doses of riboflavin is similarly promoted by concomitant food intake or by administration of anticholinergic drugs.

Levy and Jusko [13] were the first to suggest that the promotional effect of food on riboflavin absorption could be explained by slower metering out of the riboflavin from the stomach to the saturable site of riboflavin absorption in the small intestine, and they indicated that this change in the role of delivery of the vitamin would allow more efficient absorption.

In my studies, I have shown that the absorption of pharmacologic doses of riboflavin is enhanced by dietary fiber, particularly coarse bran. Riboflavin is also more efficiently absorbed when given with a glucose polymer rather than with milk [14].

The absorption of the antifungal drug griseofulvin is specifically enhanced by intake with meals containing fat. Since griseofulvin is a highly lipid-soluble drug, it has been suggested that the fat can dissolve the drug or perhaps that the intake of fat with food promotes release of bile, which also increases absorption of this drug [15,16].

Prior to the time when ultramicronized preparations of griseofulvin became available, I observed that in elderly diabetics or elderly patients with peripheral vascular disease who had extensive fungus infections of the lower limbs, the therapeutic response to griseofulvin was poor and that this impairment of therapeutic response could be explained by the fat restriction of the patient's diet. When the drug was given with a small amount of corn oil, its therapeutic efficacy was restored.

Melander [7] has emphasized that food effects on drug absorption are not always of clinical importance. Studies carried out to show these effects have been conducted using a single meal. However, what is important in clinical practice is whether with drug schedules involving repeated doses, the ther-

Table 5-1
Drugs for Which Absorption is Influenced by Food

Drugs whose absorption is reduced by food
Ampicillin
Penicillin V suspension
Penicillin G suspension
Cephalexin suspension
Nafcillin tablets
Tetracycline capsules
Erythromycin stearate film-coated tablets
Aspirin tablets
Levodopa
Methyldopa
Isoniazid
Rifampin
Drugs whose absorption is delayed by food
Cephalexin capsules
Cephalexin suspension
Cefaclor capsules
Metronidazole tablets
Aspirin tablets
Digoxin tablets
Cimetidine
Drugs whose absorption is enhanced by food
Erythromycin ethylsuccinate suspension
Erythromycin estolate capsules
Nitrofurantoin tablets
Propranolol
Hydrochlorothiazide tablets
Metoprolol
Dicumarol tablets
Diazepam tablets
Griseofulvin tablets

apeutic range of drug in the blood and tissues is reached but not exceeded. Drugs such as tetracycline, which are inefficiently absorbed irrespective of food and are much less well absorbed when taken with foods containing calcium or magnesium need to be prescribed away from eating times in order that therapeutic blood levels may be attained.

Food effects on drug absorption are summarized in Table 5-1.

Effects of Drugs on Nutrient Absorption

Many drugs have been shown to reduce nutrient absorption as a result of either intraluminal interaction, drug-induced mucosal damage, or drug-induced maldigestion. Primary drug-induced malabsorption occurs when the

Table 5–2
Drugs That Cause Primary Malabsorption

Drug	*Usage*	*Malabsorption or Fecal Nutrient Loss*	*Mechanism*
Mineral oil	Laxative	Carotene, vitamins A, D, K	Physical barrier, nutrients dissolve in mineral oil and are lost; micelle formation decreased
Phenolphthalein	Laxative	Vitamin D, Ca	Intestinal hurry; K depletion; loss of structural integrity
Neomycin	Antibiotic to "sterilize" gut	Fat, nitrogen, Na, K, Ca, Fe, lactose, sucrose, vitamin B_{12}	Structural defect; pancreatic lipase lowered; binding of bile salts (acids)
Cholestyramine	Hypercholesterolemic agents, bile acid sequestrants	Fat, vitamins A, K, folate	Binding of bile acids (salts) and nutrients
Colestipol	Hypercholesterolemic agents, bile acid sequestrants	Fat, vitamins A, K, folate	Binding of bile acids (salts) and nutrients
Potassium chloride	Potassium repletion	Vitamin B_{12}	Ileal pH lowered
Colchicine	Antiinflammatory agent in gout	Fat, carotene, Na, K, vitamin B_{12}, lactose intolerance	Mitotic arrest; structural defect; enzyme damage
Sulfasalazine	Antiinflammatory agent in ulcerative colitis and regional enteritis	Folacin	Mucosal block in folate uptake
Methyldopa	Antihypertensive agent	Folacin, vitamin B_{12}, iron	Autoimmune mechanism?

Table 5-3
Drugs Causing Secondary Malabsorption

Drug	*Usage*	*Malabsorption*	*Mechanism*
Prednisone (other glucocorticoids)	In allergic and collagen disease	Calcium	Calcium transport ↓
Phenobarbital	Anticonvulsant	Calcium	Impaired metabolism of vitamin D
Phenytoin	Anticonvulsant	Calcium	Impaired metabolism of vitamin D
Primidone	Anticonvulsant	Calcium	Impaired metabolism of vitamin D
Glutethimide	Sedative	Calcium	Impaired Ca transport
Methotrexate	Leukemia	Calcium	Acute folacin deficiency

drug effect occurs directly and without an intermediate nutrient-nutrient interaction. Examples of primary drug-induced malabsorption are given in Table 5-2.

Secondary drug-induced malabsorption occurs when the drug affects the availability of a nutrient which is required to facilitate absorption of a second nutrient—for example, phenytoin may interfere with vitamin D metabolism so that calcium absorption is decreased [17]. Methotrexate can cause secondary malabsorption because the drug induces acute folate deficiency, and this deficiency causes changes in the intestinal mucosa which reduce the absorption of other nutrients. Table 5-3 shows drugs that induce secondary malabsorption.

Primary drug-induced malabsorption may be commoner in older patients because they are more likely to consume the drugs that have direct effects on drug absorption. Two classes of over-the-counter drugs taken by the elderly, antacids and laxatives, can cause primary malabsorption. On the other hand, secondary malabsorption may be more common in children because children with seizure disorders are given anticonvulsant drugs such as phenytoin and phenobarbital, and children with acute lymphoblastic leukemia receive methotrexate.

Cimetidine is a drug now in common use that may affect absorptive capacity. It is currently considered the drug of choice in the management of duodenal ulcers, the Zollinger-Ellison syndrome, systemic mastocytosis, and the multiple endocrine adenoma syndrome. It has been of particular concern that cimetidine, in addition to inhibiting gastric acid secretion, could reduce secretion of the gastric intrinsic factor. While it has been reported by some investigators that cimetidine decreases secretion of intrinsic factor in response to pentagastrin stimulation, findings have varied; it is now generally agreed that the effects of cimetidine on intrinsic factor secretion are small and should not cause concern that the amount of intrinsic factor production might be insufficient for the formation of the intrinsic factor–vitamin B_{12} complex necessary for vitamin B_{12} absorption. Although there is little concern that vitamin B_{12} malabsorption could occur with intake of cimetidine because of reduced gastric intrinsic factor secretion, it has been shown that cimetidine reduces the absorption of food-bound vitamin B_{12}, probably because of the combined effects of decreased secretion of intrinsic factor and decreased secretion of gastric acid. In patients who need to take cimetidine over long periods, the vitamin B_{12} status should be monitored regularly so that vitamin B_{12} can be administered if serum levels of the vitamin become reduced. It seems that the major effect of the cimetidine on vitamin B_{12} absorption occurs because the drug slows the gastric release of vitamin B_{12} from animal protein foods [18].

While there is a risk of inducing vitamin B_{12} malabsorption with continued intake of cimetidine, this drug is also being used to promote absorption under special circumstances. Several authors have shown that cimetidine improves digestive capacity in patients with pancreatic insufficiency when the drug is used with oral pancreatic enzyme supplements [19–21]. The idea that cimetidine would benefit patients with pancreatic insufficiency when given with pancreatic enzymes was based on the concept that if gastric acid output were decreased in these patients, it would limit gastric inactivation of the orally administered pancreatic enzyme preparation and would also allow greater recovery of enzyme activity in the duodenum [22]. While early studies of the effectiveness of cimetidine in the management of maldigestion in patients with pancreatic insufficiency were very short, a study by Hubbard and colleagues was of longer duration [23]. These authors studied the effectiveness of cimetidine as an adjunct therapy to pancreatic enzymes in eight patients with cystic fibrosis who had evidence of pancreatic insufficiency. Cimetidine was given in a dose of 300 mg, three times a day, for a six-week period. Patients showed an increase in weight and a decrease in steatorrhea. No side effects were encountered.

A further evaluation of the usefulness of cimetidine in the long-term management of such patients clearly needs to be carried out. In patients with pancreatic insufficiency secondary to chronic alcoholic pancreatitis, neither cimetidine nor antacids improve digestive capacity when pancreatic enzyme replacements are given [24].

Indications and contraindications for the use of cimetidine in patients with pancreatic insufficiency, as in other patients, have to be carefully evaluated, not only because of the possible adverse effect of the drug on vitamin B_{12} absorption but also because cimetidine is known to be a potent inhibitor of drug metabolism [25,26]. Slowing of drug metabolism could have serious effects in elderly patients with impaired liver or kidney function.

Drug-Food and Drug-Alcohol Incompatibilities

Acute reactions following drug-food or drug-alcohol incompatibilities can be life-threatening or so unpleasant as to reduce drug compliance. Drug-food incompatibilities that are life-threatening include the tyramine reaction, which may follow ingestion of foods of high tyramine content by patients taking drugs that are monamine oxidase (MAO) inhibitors. Antidepressant drugs that are MAO-inhibitors have long been known to induce hypertensive crises when patients consume foods high in monamines, such as tyramine and dopamine. These foods include aged cheeses, pickled herrings, chicken livers, Chianti wines, and broad beans. Inhibition of monamine metabolism in patients taking these drugs triggers the release of catecholamines, which explains the acute hypertensive attacks. It has been reported more recently by Kent-Smith and Durack that patients receiving isoniazid develop tyramine reactions [27]. Procarbazine, which is used in the treatment of Hodgkin's disease, can also cause tyramine reactions, though the severity is not as great as with the MAO-inhibiting antidepressant drugs [28,29].

Alcohol ingestion evokes an adverse reaction in patients receiving several different drugs. Metronidazole (Flagyl), which is used as the drug of choice in *Trichomonas* vaginitis, intestinal amebiasis, giardiasis, as a preventive of infection after colon surgery, and to a limited extent as a radiation sensitizer in cancer patients, produces an intolerance to alcohol. The alcohol-metronidazole reaction is similar to that which occurs with disulfiram (Antabuse). Alcohol intolerance with a disulfiram-like reaction has also been observed in patients taking cephalosporin antibiotics [30,31].

Acute adverse reactions to alcohol with development of flushing may also occur in patients receiving calcium carbimide, furazolidone, griseofulvin, quinacrine, chloramphenicol, phentolamine, and also certain oral antidiabetic agents including chlorpropamide [32].

Facial flushing after intake of alcoholic beverages has been estimated to occur in 13–33 percent of insulin-independent diabetics taking the sulfonylurea drug chlorpropamide [33]. In 1978 Leslie and Pike developed a single challenge test for the chlorpropamide-alcohol flush (CPAF) reaction, in which 40 ml of sherry was given 12 hours after a single 250-mg dose of chlorpropamide. These authors not only found a high degree of correlation between flushing with this test and a clinical history of flushing after intake of alcoholic beverages in patients taking chlorpropamide (33 out of 35 patients), they also found that a positive flush reaction with this test occurred much more frequently in non-insulin-independent diabetics than in insulin-dependent diabetics or nondiabetics [34]. Subsequently these authors and others in the same group found that a positive flush reaction was more common in a subgroup of diabetics who displayed a lower susceptibility to diabetic retinopathy, ischemic heart disease, and peripheral vascular disease [35,36].

Since then, this drug-alcohol incompatibility has come to be used as a diagnostic test for this subtype of insulin-independent diabetes [37]. However, the sensitivity and specificity of the test have been called in doubt by a study of DeSilva and colleagues [38]. These investigators tested 50 insulin-independent diabetics with the CPAF single challenge test. Nine of these diabetics also flushed when a placebo was given instead of chlorpropamide. Also in a control group of 21 nondiabetics, two showed the so-called specific CPAF reaction.

Drug-food and drug-alcohol incompatibilities are summarized in Table 5-4.

Table 5–4
Drug-Nutrient and Drug-Alcohol Incompatibilities

Classification	*Reactant 1*	*Reactant 2*	*Effect*
Tyramine reactions	MAO inhibitors Antidepressants (e.g., phenelzine) Procarbazine Isoniazid (INH, isonicotine hydrazine)	High tyramine/dopamine foods Cheese Red wines Chicken liver Broad beans	Flushing Hypertension Cerebrovascular accidents
Disulfiram reactions	Aldehyde dehydrogenase inhibitors Disulfiram (Antabuse) Calcium carbimide Metronidazole Nitrofurantoin Sulfonylureas	Ethanol Beer Wine Liquor Foods containing alcohol	Flushing, headache Nausea, vomiting Chest and abdominal pain
Hypoglycemic reactions	Insulin releasers Oral hypoglycemic agents Sugar (as in sweet mixes)	Ethanol	Weakness Mental confusion Irrational behavior Loss of consciousness
Flush reactions[a]	Miscellaneous Chlorpropamide (in diabetics) Griseofulvin Tetrachloroethylene	Ethanol	Flush Dyspnea Headache

[a]See Pierpaoli [2].

Problems of Noncompliance in Relation to Drug-Nutrient Interactions

It is well recognized that noncompliance with prescribed medication is a serious problem, especially when noncompliance has potentially serious outcomes. Dirks and Kinsman emphasized that among the types of noncompliance, underusage and erratic usage of drugs are common. Though underusage reduces the risk of serious drug toxicity, it occurs at the expense of therapeutic efficacy [39].

I am concerned that drug-nutrient interactions, and particularly drug-nutrient and drug-alcohol incompatibilities, may reduce medication compliance because of the aversive responses to drug intake. There is a real need for education of physicians and patients about drug-nutrient interactions to emphasize the risk of noncompliance with prescribed medication as an outcome of drug-related reactions to food or alcohol. Prescriptions should bear clear instructions as to when medications should be taken in relation to food. This will help only if the patient understands the instructions so that drugs better taken fasting are actually taken fasting, and drugs better taken after food are taken after food. Similarly, it is important that physicians as well as pharmacists, nurses, and dietitians be familiar with the concepts of drug-induced malabsorption and know that many forms of drug-induced malabsorption occur because drugs are taken close to eating time.

Finally, patients should be adequately warned about the possibility of drug-food and drug-alcohol incompatibilities. Some side effects of drugs have to be endured because the beneficial therapeutic effects of the drug outweigh the side effects; nevertheless, it is unnecessary for patients to have to endure reactions, such as flush reactions, which could easily be avoided. Health care professionals may be persuaded that these reactions are commonly the patient's fault, but they are usually the fault of the prescriber who forgets to give adequate warnings.

Summary

Food can affect the absorption of drugs; drugs can affect the absorption of nutrients; and both food and alcohol can evoke acute adverse drug reactions when taken with drugs. Certain drugs are better absorbed when taken fasting and others are better absorbed when taken with food. Recent advances in knowledge of the mechanisms by which food influences drug absorption have been discussed, including selected examples of drugs for which absorption is retarded, reduced, or enhanced by food. The net effects of these drug-food interactions are of clinical importance when feeding or abstention from food at the time of drug intake influences whether therapeutic levels of the drug are attained in the blood.

Drug-induced malabsorption has been discussed, with emphasis on newer knowledge of drugs most likely to produce such adverse drug reactions in patients at special risk.

Flush reactions have been described which are examples of drug-food or drug-alcohol incompatibility.

Overall focus has been on outcomes of drug-food or drug-alcohol interactions which may lead to a reduction in drug efficacy, to an increase in drug toxicity or to a lessening of drug compliance. Means of prevention of unwanted drug-food or drug-alcohol interactions have been proposed which involve special patient instruction on appropriate drug usage.

References

1. Welling, P.G. Influence of food and diet on gastrointestinal drug absorption: A review. *J. Pharmacokinet. Biopharm.* 5:291–334, 1977.

2. Pierpaoli, P.G. Drug therapy and diet. *Drug Intel. Clin. Pharm.* 6:89–99, 1972.

3. Roholt, K., Nielsen, B., Kristensen, E. Clinical pharmacology of pivampicillin. *Antimicrob. Agents Chemother.* 6:563–571, 1974.

4. Neuvonen, P.J. Interactions with the absorption of tetracyclines. *Drugs* 11:45–54, 1976.

5. Melander, A., Danielson, K., Hanson, A., et al. Reduction of isoniazid bioavailability in normal men by concomitant intake of food. *Acta Med. Scand.* 200:93–97, 1976.

6. Acocella, G. Clinical pharmacokinetics of rifampicin. *Clin. Pharmacokinet.* 3:108–127, 1978.

7. Melander, A. Food intake and drug bioavailability. In Harper, A.E., Davis, G.K. (Eds.), *Nutrition in Health and Disease and International Development: Symposia from the Twelfth International Congress of Nutrition.* New York: Alan R. Liss, 1981. Pp. 747–756.

8. Hurwitz, A. Antacid therapy and drug kinetics. *Clin. Pharmacokinet.* 2:269–280, 1977.

9. Hurwitz, A., Schlozman, D.L. Effects of antacids on gastrointestinal absorption of isoniazid in rat and man. *Am. Rev. Respir. Dis.* 109:41–47, 1974.

10. Melander, A., Wahlin, E. Enhancement of dicoumarol bioavailability by concomitant food intake. *Eur. J. Clin. Pharmacol.* 14:441–444, 1978.

11. Melander, A., Brante, G., Johansson, O., et al. Influence of food on the absorption of phenytoin in man. *Eur. J. Clin. Pharmacol.* 15:269–274, 1979.

12. Beermann, B., Groschinsky-Grin, D.M. Enhancement of the gastrointestinal absorption of hydrochlorothiazide by propantheline. *Eur. J. Clin. Pharmacol.* 13:385–387, 1978.

13. Levy, G., Jusko, W.J. Factors affecting the absorption of riboflavin in man. *J. Pharm. Sci.* 55:285–289, 1966.

14. Roe, D.A. Intergroup and intragroup variables affecting interpretation of studies of drug effects of nutritional status. In Harper, A.E., Davis, G.K. (Eds.), *Nutrition in Health and Disease and International Development: Symposia from the Twelfth International Congress of Nutrition.* New York: Alan R. Liss, 1981. Pp. 757–771.

15. Crounse, R.G. Human pharmacology of griseofulvin: The effect of fat intake on gastrointestinal absorption. *J. Invest. Dermatol.* 37:529–533, 1961.

16. Kabasakalian, P., Katz, M., Rosenkrantz, B., Townley, E. Parameters affecting absorption of griseofulvin in a human subject using urinary metabolic excretion data. *J. Pharm. Sci.* 59:595–600, 1970.

17. Zerwekh, J.E., Hanan, R., Tindall, R., Pak., C.Y.C. Decreased serum 24,25-dihydroxyvitamin D concentration during long-term anticonvulsant therapy in adult epileptics. *Ann. Neurol.* 12:184–186, 1982.

18. McGuigan, J.E. A consideration of the adverse effects of cimetidine. *Gastroenterology* 80:181–192, 1980.

19. Regan, P.T., Malagelada, J., diMagno, E.P., et al. Comparative effects of antacids, cimetidine and enteric coating on the therapeutic response to oral enzymes in severe pancreatic insufficiency. *N. Engl. J. Med.* 297:854–858, 1977.

20. Cox, K.L., Isenberg, J.N., Osher, A.B., Dooley, R.R. The effect of cimetidine on maldigestion in cystic fibrosis. *J. Pediatr.* 94:488–492, 1979.

21. Bianchi-Porro, G., Dolcini, R., Grossi, E., et al. Cimetidine in treatment of pancreatic insufficiency. *Lancet* 2:878–879, 1979.

22. Finkelstein, W., Isselbacher, K.J. Drug therapy: Cimetidine. *N. Engl. J. Med.* 299:922–926, 1978.

23. Hubbard, V.S., Dewey Dunn, G., Lester, L.A. Effectiveness of cimetidine as an adjunct to supplemental pancreatic enzymes in patients with cystic fibrosis. *Am. J. Clin. Nutr.* 33:2281–2286, 1980.

24. Graham, D.Y. Pancreatic enzyme replacement. The effect of antacids or cimetidine. *Dig. Dis. Sci.* 27:485–491, 1982.

25. Knodell, R.G., Holtzman, J.L., Crankshaw, D.L., et al. Hepatic metabolism by rat and human hepatic microsomes in response to interaction with H^2-receptor antagonists. *Gastroenterology* 82:4–88, 1982.

26. Speeg, K.V., Patwardhan, R.V., Avant, G.R., et al. Inhibition of microsomal drug metabolism by histamine H_2-receptor antagonists studied in vivo and in vitro in rodents. *Gastroenterology* 82:89–96, 1982.

27. Kent-Smith, C., Durack, D.T. Isoniazid and reactions to cheese. *Ann. Intern. Med.* 88:520–521, 1978.

28. Spivack, S.D. Procarbazine. *Ann. Intern. Med.* 81:795–800, 1974.

29. Roe, D.A. Drug-nutrient interactions. *Med. Clin. North Am.* 63:985–1007, 1979.

30. Goldman, P. Metronidazole. *N. Engl. J. Med.* 303:1212–1218, 1980.

31. Reeves, D.S., Davies, A.J. Antabuse effect with cephalosporins. *Lancet* 2:540, 1980.

32. Seixas, F. Alcohol and its drug interaction. *Ann. Intern. Med.* 83:86–92, 1975.

33. Fitzgerald, M.G., Gaddie, R., Malins, J.M., et al. Alcohol sensitivity in diabetics receiving chlorpropamide. *Diabetes* 11:40–43, 1962.

34. Leslie, R.D.G., Pike, D.A. Chlorpropamide alcohol flushing: A dominantly inherited trait associated with diabetes. *Br. Med. J.* 2:1519–1521, 1978.

35. Leslie, R.D.G., Barnett, A.H., Pike, D.A. Chlorpropamide alcohol flushing and diabetic retinopathy. *Lancet* 1:997–999, 1979.

36. Barnett, A.H., Pike, D.A. Chlorpropamide alcohol flushing and large vessel disease in non-insulin dependent diabetes. *Br. Med. J.* 281:261–262, 1980.

37. Cobberling, J., Bengsch, N., Bruggeboes, B., et al. The chlorpropamide alcohol flush. *Diabetologia* 19:359–363, 1980.

38. DeSilva, N.E., Tunbridge, W.M.G., Alberti, K.G.M.M. Low incidence of chlorpropamide alcohol flushing in diet-treated non-insulin dependent diabetes. *Lancet* 1:128–131, 1981.

39. Dirks, J.F., Kinsman, R.A. Non-dichotomous patterns of medication usage: The yes-no fallacy. *Clin. Pharmacol. Ther.* 31:413–417, 1982.

6 Diet in the Epidemiology of Cancer

Saxon Graham, Ph.D.

It is likely that agents exogenous to an organism may either enhance or reduce the likelihood that it will develop disease. Such exogenous agents may gain access to the organism via the emotions, the skin, the respiratory system, or the alimentary system. Thus, consideration of diet must figure importantly in studies of epidemiology, and specifically in the epidemiology of cancer at various sites. The hypotheses linking diet and cancer are many. Those that link the ingestion of meats or fats to increased risk of a variety of cancers, notably those of the colon and breast, are important.

Among the hypotheses dealing with vegetables is that ingestion of fiber will reduce the risk of cancer of the colon. In addition, a number of hypotheses, mainly devolving from studies of cell cultures and of carcinogenesis in animals, link the various antioxidants and particularly vitamin C to reduced risk of cancer. Another class of nutrients that has been found in animal studies to reduce the risk specifically of colon cancer includes compounds found in the cruciferous vegetables, such as cabbage, brussels sprouts, broccoli, cauliflower, and the like. A few epidemiologic studies of cancer patients and controls seem to corroborate this finding. Finally, studies using both cell cultures and animals have found a substantial inhibition of tumor growth in tissue challenged with known carcinogens and treated by either vitamin A or synthetic retinoids. Here again, there are a few epidemiologic studies of diet in human patients and controls that appear to provide corroboration of the experimental findings.

Although it would appear that there is a growing mass of data linking various food substances to reduced risk of a variety of cancers, and almost none linking vegetable substances to enhanced risk, there are sufficient difficulties with the methods of all the various types of studies to make the findings less than fully convincing. In general, there are a certain number of corroborative findings, but the potential for bias in the methodology of these studies makes it necessary to conduct substantial further research not only on the hypotheses but in some cases in methodology.

This research was supported by NIH grant CA11535.

Methods

Researchers have used a number of methods to study diet. One of these has been to infer ingestion of various nutrients from the study of blood, urine, feces, or other materials of patients after they have been diagnosed as compared with controls. From such findings, inferences might be made as to the kinds of diet that might have produced the disease. Studies have shown a correlation between the amount of fats ingested and the appearance of bile acids in the feces and of vitamin C and its appearance in the urine. But as with all approaches in this difficult area, there are certain drawbacks. The patient's disease may have substantially altered the fashion in which dietary factors are transformed in the alimentary system. The therapy for the disease could also alter the metabolic effects. Moreover, certain dietary components involved in current hypotheses of cancer etiology may be influenced by variations in individual metabolism and other factors. For example, the microbial content and activity of the gut have been observed to vary with changing levels of psychological or physical stress, as well as with changes in diet. Similarly, although the amount of blood cholesterol may be lowered by manipulating diet in the clinical situation, the level of blood cholesterol observed in a cross-sectional study may also be the product of other factors such as psychological or physical stress and may not reflect diet alone. Thus, attempts to infer diet from the characteristics of materials from patients and controls may involve some error. Another drawback is the high cost of this approach and the difficulty in getting materials from enough patients and controls to do adequate statistical and especially multivariate analyses. On the other hand, used prospectively, given the prodigious amounts of time and money needed, follow-up on persons with high and low blood cholesterol levels in numerous studies has unequivocally associated high cholesterol levels with a high risk of coronary heart disease [1–4]. On diseases of lower incidence, such as cancer, the method will be even more expensive.

Attempts to generalize from animal to human disease are also fraught with difficulty. There are many instances in which conclusions drawn on the basis of studies of animals do not hold up in studying humans. For example, DDT may be carcinogenic to animals, but it has not been shown to be so in humans. We have numerous animal studies indicating that saccharin is associated with cancer, but a number of epidemiologic studies of human bladder cancer patients and controls, some with very substantial numbers and methodology, indicate no risk associated with the use of nonnutritive sweeteners [5,6]. Two studies do, but, strangely, only for males [7,8]. Our large-scale study shows no increase in risk with increases in ingestion of saccharin. No one has been able to produce cancer in animals with alcohol; in fact, Fred Bock of Roswell Park Memorial Institute has found tumor inhibition in mice painted with moderate amounts of bourbon (personal communication).

However, five large epidemiologic interview studies link alcohol to oral cancer in humans [9–13]. In view of the congruence of findings in the five epidemiologic studies of humans, I would be less concerned with the lack of corroboration in animal models. Although we can discern potential pathogenicity of various factors from studies of animals, it would seem prudent, before drawing conclusions regarding human disease causation, to determine whether evidence from human epidemiology corroborates the findings from animal studies.

Some scientists have assumed that international comparisons of disease rates and food consumption patterns would provide evidence of a sort. One of the most popular of these attempts indicates that the higher the fat consumption in countries, the higher is the mortality from colon cancer. The dangers in concluding from this that high intake of dietary fats causes colon cancer are many. For one thing, considerable error may be present in the diagnosis of the cause of mortality, and indeed, for many of the countries studied, it may account for the differences observed. Thus, for example, the low mortality from colon cancer in Chili, Portugal, and Italy may be related to the fact that this internal and difficult-to-diagnose cancer may be underreported as a cause of death. Moreover, although there may be a rather high correlation indicated, the numerous exceptions are important. Thus, although Canadians and U.S. whites have the same per capita consumption of fat and oil as the Finns, Israelis, Portuguese, and Italians, they have twice the rate of colon cancer.

There are a variety of other factors that could be correlated with the mortality from colon cancer in such an international comparison. Higginson has shown that as the industrialization of countries increases, so do colon cancer rates, and we could hypothesize with some confidence that per capita consumption of refined carbohydrates, expensive garden vegetables, and aspirin, not to mention air pollution and number of telephones, cars, and refrigerators per capita, might also characterize nations with high colon cancer rates as compared to those with low rates [14].

Most important, inferring fat consumption of patients from an average for the nation may be faulty. There is good evidence that in the more industrialized nations, the diet is quite heterogeneous from individual to individual. It is obviously impossible to generalize from an average rate of fat consumption based on the millions of people in a society to the comparative few who develop colon cancer. There is no evidence on the fat consumption of the colon cancer patients themselves; they may be very different from the average.

When we are dealing with something as complex as diet, particularly in the developed nations, it would seem that one logical and inexpensive method would be to query patients and controls about what they eat. Useful methods have been the diet diary, statements as to usual diet, the 24-hour recall of foods eaten, and the frequency with which various specific foods are eaten. The prime difficulty here is the possibility of error in recollection of amounts and frequencies of various foods eaten, especially over the extended period necessary when diseases of long latency are studied.

A number of studies of the reliability of the food frequency interviews have been conducted, most on small numbers of subjects. Dawber and colleagues [15], Nomura and associates [16], Reshef and Epstein [17], and my colleagues and I [18] compared results of diet interviews carried on at two different times and found an average error of less than 15 percent, which varied by type of food [15–18].

In our Western New York Interview Study of Diet and Cancer, we are comparing all patients with neighborhood controls in the three most populous counties. We have built into the research a variety of quality control procedures, including the diet diary and the 24-hour recall. Another approach is to compare spouses' reports of the patients' frequency of ingestion of various foods. Our findings, like those of Kolonel in a similar study [19], indicate an amount of spouse agreement on frequency of food ingestion consistent with levels found in the studies described in the previous paragraph.

Of course, a comparison of spouse estimates of the frequency with which one of them eats a given item, or a reinterview with a specific individual, does not examine the extent to which the report represents actual fact. Nevertheless, it is likely that the fact, as suggested by the validity studies of Jain, Hankin, and others, may lie somewhere near the two estimates provided. For example, in an English study, entries on a seven-day diet diary kept by subjects in the British National Food Survey were compared with estimates derived from 63 Cambridgeshire subjects who were instructed by a nutritionist on how to weigh and record everything ingested and who were later visited several times to check on the accuracy of the weighing [20]. It is interesting that the total dietary fiber was 19.9 g per day for this study group, as compared with 19.7 g per day for the National Food Survey. Madden and Gersovitz [21] observed 74 people in a congregate feeding program in Pennsylvania and compared what they saw the people eating with data from interviews conducted the next day. They warn that although there may be false-negative results, they regard the interview procedure useful as a method.

These studies do not consider the problem of recall of diet over the period necessary to study diseases of long latency, such as cancer. Essentially, all the findings of studies of diet and cancer are predicated on stability of diet throughout life, and we now have little evidence that this is true. It is possible, however, that lifetime diet patterns are set at a young age, that there is consistency in dietary patterns of individuals throughout life, and that the diet recalled for the period before symptom onset is similar to that 20 years earlier, or similar enough to distinguish large groups of patients from controls. Of course, one way around this problem is to query a large number of people on their diet and then follow them for many years to see whether incidence of disease differs by diet. Hirayama, Bjelke, and my colleagues and I are in the process of doing this. In any event, it is true that the results of diet interview studies have often been consistent with those of experiments with animal models and organ cultures.

We can conclude that there are a number of drawbacks to the various methods of study—the use of animals, study of biologic materials from humans, and interviews. Nevertheless, it is also true that numerous findings on the various hypotheses of etiology have accumulated, some replicated, some not, some congruent with findings in other fields and some not. These findings will be discussed in the following sections.

The Animal Fats Hypothesis

Reddy and Wynder hypothesized that increases in dietary fats are accompanied by increases in bile acids and neutral steroids and bacteria in the feces which could metabolize them into carcinogenic substances possibly related to methylcholanthrene [22]. There is some evidence supporting this hypothesis. For example, Reddy examined 8 individuals who first were on a high-meat diet and then on a no-meat diet, 12 so-called vegetarians, and 11 Seventh Day Adventist vegetarians, comparing each of these groups with healthy omnivorous people [23]. A similar study was accomplished by Aries and colleagues of 15 Vegans, members of an English group who eat no animal products [24]. They found that the concentration of bile acids in feces of the vegetarians ranged from 21 to 86 percent of that of the omnivores, and the concentration of neutral steroids from 33 to 82 percent. On the other hand, Cummings found no increase in bile acid in men on a high-meat diet [25]. Recently Reddy and Wynder have compared colon cancer patients versus controls as to fecal neutral steroid and bile acid concentrations, and they found significantly larger concentrations in the cancer patients [22]. In addition, animals challenged with dimethylhydrazine and fed either vegetable oil or beef fat exhibited more tumors than animals on a control diet. It would appear that the evidence is accumulating that a high-fat diet might indeed produce conditions in the gut conducive to the manufacture of powerful carcinogens. However, there are several cautions to be observed: (1) findings with animals are not necessarily applicable to humans; (2) studies of excretions of societal groups, such as the Seventh Day Adventists, tell nothing of the characteristics of patients and controls; and (3) studies of excretions of cancer patients and controls are inconclusive because whatever differences are found may be the result of the development of their cancer or the treatment of it rather than a preexisting situation that produced the cancer.

A fair number of studies have compared colon cancer patients and controls as to their dietary habits prior to diagnosis of their disease, as reported in interviews. To date, one such study supports the meats hypothesis—that by

Haenszel, in a series of 179 patients and 357 controls from Hawaii [26]. So does another from Toronto; but a number of studies have found no difference in the ingestion of meats by cancer patients and controls. This is true of a new study by Haenszel of the Japanese in Japan [27], as well as studies by Wynder in New York [28], Higginson in the Midwest [14], and my colleagues and I in Buffalo, New York [29]. Bjelke found negative results for all meats except processed meats [30]. Our case-control study at Roswell Park Memorial Institute showed a decrease in risk of colon cancer with increases in meat eating [31]. John Cummings, of Cambridge University, in his initial analyses also found a decrease in risk with increases in protein ingested in a study in Scandinavia (personal communication). And the results of a number of prospective studies of serum cholesterol are consistent. Each involves many thousands of people studied for many years: three large studies in Chicago [1], one in Puerto Rico [2], one in Framingham, Massachusetts [3], and one in Yugoslavia [4]. These studies do not support the hypothesis that high serum cholesterol increases the risk of cancer; rather, in most of them, the opposite seems true. Serum cholesterol is affected to some degree by diet, and it is reasonable to conclude on the basis of these findings that we have little epidemiologic support for the proposition that high-fat diets increase the risk of cancer in humans.

The Fiber Hypothesis

The fiber hypothesis as it relates to the etiology of colon cancer is based on a simple and logical-sounding theory. It maintains that a high-fiber diet can result in a shorter time for material to pass through the gut. This presumably reduces the opportunity for bacteria in the bowel to produce a carcinogen and reduces the opportunity for the carcinogen to work on the gut wall. In addition, the high-fiber diet increases the total bulk of the content so that any carcinogenic materials passing through do so in a more dilute form. Eastwood and Burkitt [32,33] furnished some evidence for a dilution effect. But there is disagreement in the literature on many of these points. No one has come up with unequivocal evidence that high fiber always shortens transit time. It is possible to cite studies on both sides of the issue.

A few studies have been conducted on the effects of dietary fiber using experimentally induced colon cancer in animals, with equivocal results. Fleiszer [34] showed a reduction in tumor incidence upon administration of fiber; Ward [35], Wilson [36], and Cruse [37] showed no effect; and Asp, in another study, found an enhanced incidence [38].

On the epidemiologic level, there have been few studies. Burkitt [39] cites a study comparing ingestion of fiber with transit times in English and African boarding school boys. He found that Africans eat more fiber, have shorter transit times, and have less colon cancer. In later studies of occupational groups in England and Africa, his findings were similar. One should note that he did not study cases and controls but merely generalized from entire societies to the few individuals who develop colon cancer. One epidemiologic case-control interview study, conducted by Modan and colleagues [40] on populations in Israel, suggests a low risk of colon cancer for individuals who frequently eat fibrous foods. These researchers compared 198 patients with age- and sex-matched hospitalized and neighborhood controls. In generating their findings, they grouped a large number of foods containing no less than 0.5 percent fiber. They found that the only group of foods the patients ate less of than the controls was the fibrous group. John Cummings has observed similar findings in four Scandinavian populations (personal communication). In San Francisco, Dales and associates [41] studied the reported dietary habits of 77 black patients with colorectal cancer and 215 matched controls. Colon cancer patients were found not to differ from controls on fats or fiber studied separately. It is interesting, however, that individuals with both a high-fat and a low-fiber diet had a risk of 2.68 relative to those with a low-fat, high-fiber diet ($p<0.05$). Bjelke found that the risk of colon cancer declined slightly with increases in consumption of fibrous foods [30]. Some other studies by Higginson and Haenszel [14,27] fail to support the link between vegetables or fibrous foods and colon cancer.

In short, there are a few findings that support the fiber hypothesis in the etiology of colon cancer, but few are uncontradicted. However, fruits and vegetables not only contribute fiber to the diet but account for nearly all of the typical intake of vitamin C, two-thirds of that of vitamin A, substantial amounts of vitamin E, and contain numerous chemicals having antioxidant or other potential cancer-inhibition properties.

Role of Vitamins in Cancer Epidemiology

Vitamin C

The attribution of a protective effect from fruit and vegetable consumption to the vitamin C that these sources may contain stems mainly from evidence that formation of carcinogenic nitrosamines can be inhibited by vitamin C. Little actual epidemiologic evidence indentifies vitamin C as a specific quality of fruit and vegetable consumption accounting for any risk reduction [26]. Bjelke [30], in the aforementioned studies in Norway and the United States, found that gastric and colon cancer patients reported lower intake of vitamin C when measured by an index aggregating the vitamin C content of various foods by the frequency of their consumption. He also found the risk of gastric cancer to be less for those ingesting large amounts of vegetables. Sorenson and Lyon, in an unpublished report on the basis of extensive dietary interviewing of 300 colon cancer patients and 600 age-matched controls, found that the nondisease persons reported significantly higher than usual intake of vitamin C than the cancer patients.

My colleagues and I had similar findings for cancer of the larynx in a study based on interviews with about 370 patients and controls at Roswell Park Institute [42]. We found an increased risk with decreases in amount of vitamin C ingested. Use of tobacco and alcohol increase the risk of cancer of the larynx, so it was interesting to observe that there is a risk reduction with each increase in vitamin C when adjusted statistically for smoking, alcohol, and both factors together. It would appear that vitamin C is a factor to be studied in future inquiries.

Vitamin A

Several laboratory investigations, both animal and in vitro studies, have shown tumor inhibition by vitamin A in its various forms. Saffiotti and colleagues [43] treated Syrian golden hamsters with a series of intratracheal instillations of the carcinogen benzo(a)pyrene (BP). Half of the animals were then fed 5 mg of vitamin A palmitate in corn oil by stomach tube twice weekly. The vitamin A group experienced a marked reduction in the incidence of respiratory tumors, particularly squamous tumors, and a reduction of squamous metaplasia. A lower incidence of tumors at nonrespiratory sites was also observed. Others have come up with similar findings.

Chu and Malmgren inhibited the induction of squamous cell carcinomas of the hamster uterine cervix by dimethylbenz(a)anthracene (DMBA) with vitamin A palmitate supplementation of the diet [44]. In a related study, Nettesheim and Williams demonstrated inhibition of metaplastic lung nodules by all-transretinyl acetate when rats with no symptoms of vitamin deficiency and adequate liver stores of vitamin A were challenged by 3-methylcholanthrene [45].

Newberne and Suphakarn reported enhanced inhibition of dimethylhydrazine-induced colon tumors by one of the synthetic retinoids, 13-*cis* retinoic acid, even when diets of control animals were amply supplemented by retinyl acetate [46]. Thus, different retinoids have different effects. Merriman and Bertram observed similar inhibitory properties of 13-*cis* retinoic acid in vitro. In their study of 3-methylcholanthrene-induced neoplastic transformations in cultured mouse fibroblasts, they were able to inhibit cell transformation dramatically with administration of retinyl acetate up to three weeks *after* initial treatment with the carcinogen [47].

Epidemiologic case-control interview studies furnish several instances of corroboration of these experimental findings. Hirayama [48], in a 10-year prospective study of 256,118 Japanese adults, found that people who ate larger amounts of green and yellow vegetables had lower subsequent incidence of cancer mortality from lung cancer. Lung cancer deaths among males and females, regardless of amount smoked, are elevated for those Japanese who in 1965 reported infrequent green and yellow vegetable consumption. Bjelke surveyed the dietary habits of over 8,000 Norwegian men and observed the incidence of lung cancer among them after five years. He found an index of vitamin A to be negatively associated with lung cancer incidence at all levels of cigarette smoking [49]. Note that the incidence in those with high retinoid ingestion was much lower than that in persons with less ingestion. Comparable reductions in risk have been observed in retrospective studies in Singapore [50].

Kark has utilized blood samples gathered in 1960 in Evans County, Georgia, to assess this relationship. He compared the serum retinol in blood taken from those who developed cancer at any site over the 17 years following, with that in a random sample of those who did not develop cancer. He found substantially increased risk with decreases in vitamin A [51].

Mettlin's study of 292 male lung cancer patients and 801 controls at Roswell Park Memorial Institute found significant risk reduction associated with increased amounts of dietary vitamin A, especially in heavy smokers [52]. A similar risk reduction by vitamin A intake was found in Mettlin's study of 489 cases of bladder cancer and 901 age- and sex-matched controls at Roswell Park Memorial Institute. Bladder cancer risk has long been recognized to be raised with increased cigarette smoking. When we examined the effects of increased vitamin A on bladder cancer risk, we found the risk to be reduced for heavy smokers, light smokers, and nonsmokers [53].

These findings prompted us to examine the dietary data we have gathered on a number of other types of patients and controls. We found that with higher vitamin A intake, risk was significantly reduced for cancer of the oral cavity [12] and the esophagus [54], controlling for the effects of other known risk factors such as cigarettes and alcohol. Our findings for cancer of the larynx [42] included a decrease in risk for increases in vitamin A ingestion. The vitamin A effect prevails when the data are adjusted for smoking, alcohol, and both factors simultaneously. It may be significant that preliminary analyses show *no* reduction in risk for vitamin A ingestion and cancer of the prostate, breast, corpus, and ovary.

We conclude that although there have been a large number of in vitro and in vivo studies and only a few human case-control studies with congruent findings, their consistency suggests the need to amplify the epidemiologic work.

Cruciferous Vegetables

Wattenberg [55] has suggested another hypothesis relating to arylhydrocarbon hydroxylase (AHH) activity in various organs of rodents. Evidence had accumulated that such activity occurs in tissues of all the major portals of entry, including the gastrointestinal tract, lung, and skin. This could represent an initial metabolic barrier to noxious chemicals in the external environment. A number of cruciferous plants, including brussels sprouts, cabbage, turnips, cauliflower, and broccoli were found to increase this activity.

Subsequently, Wattenberg [56] determined that the inducers in these vegetables are certain indoles. Later he wished to determine whether these compounds would inhibit carcinogenesis by polycyclic hydrocarbons. One of Wattenberg and Loub's experiments on the effects of indoles on the formation of DMBA-induced mammary tumors showed that when there was no indole added to the diet, 91 percent of the rats developed tumors, with an average of 1.45 tumors per rat [55]. When indole-3-carbinol and diindolylmethane were added to the diet, the proportion of animals with tumors dropped to 21 and 27 percent and the mean number of tumors dropped to 0.4. It would appear that Wattenberg has identified chemicals in cabbage, cauliflower, turnips, broccoli, and brussels sprouts which can reduce the number of tumors that appear ordinarily when animals are challenged by DMBA and BP. It may be significant that he has also inhibited tumor formation by simple feeding of these vegetables, either raw or cooked, to animals.

Our epidemiologic study [31], carried out with a primitive instrument, on a series of 196 patients and 625 controls from Roswell Park Memorial Institute showed results that are quite similar to those of Wattenberg. A decreasing frequency of eating cabbage is associated with an increased risk for cancer of the colon. There is a suggestion of a dose-response relationship. A similar dose-response relationship was encountered in analyses of two other forms of cabbage, sauerkraut and cole slaw, as well as two related vegetables, brussels sprouts and broccoli.

Some of the results of the few previous epidemiologic studies on the role of vegetables also seem consistent with our finding. Indeed, Modan [40] found that colon cancer patients consumed cabbage significantly less frequently than controls, and there was a similar directional difference for other cruciferous vegetables, such as kohlrabi, sauerkraut, turnips, and cauliflower. Bjelke's finding for vegetables in general and cabbage in particular is also congruent.

On the other hand, the studies of Haenszel and colleagues [26,27], and Higginson [14] specifically examined risk associated with various vegetables and found no interesting relationships with colon cancer. Note, too, that the relative risks for infrequent eating of cruciferous vegetables observed in our research reach only about to the level of 2 or 3. But it would be difficult to ascribe this finding to chance because of its consistency among several vegetables of the cruciferous type and because of Wattenberg's congruent findings.

The same may be said of the consistent laboratory and epidemiologic findings on vitamin A. Nevertheless, the paucity of these findings, and of those dealing with vitamins C and E, fats, and fiber, especially those on human patients and controls, testifies to the need for further inquiry. This inquiry is indeed taking place, and at a growing number of centers: Hirayama in Japan, Bjelke in Norway, Modan in Israel, Miller in Toronto. New studies in other centers will conclude in the next few years, including those by Lyon in Utah, Phillips in Los Angeles, Kolonel in Hawaii, and our own in western New York. Three prospective studies are also under way: those by Bjelke in Norway and Minnesota; ours, which deals with the New York state population; and a projected study by Hennekens and Speizer. Thus in the next few years we should have some ideas as to whether the leads uncovered so far, especially regarding vitamins A and C, fats, fiber, and cruciferous vegetables, are merely random occurrences, or whether they suggest some possibilities for the prevention of a number of different cancers.

Summary

Environmental agents, including diet, figure prominently in the epidemiology of cancer. Several methods of the study of dietary components in the epidemiology of cancer have been discussed, and a number of drawbacks pointed out. The use of animals, of biological materials from humans, and of interviews may introduce errors of interpretation in the question of association of specific dietary factors and the incidence of cancer. Several hypotheses have been advanced to link certain diets to cancer risk or to assign a mitigating role to dietary components. At present, insufficient evidence has been gathered to implicate clearly fiber, animal fats, or vitamin C or E as factors in the modulation of cancer risk. A possible, though weak, link has been suggested for cruciferous vegetables and for vitamin A in the reduction of risk of cancer. Several studies are currently under way which should provide answers in the next several years on whether vitamin A and C, fats, fiber, and the cruciferous vegetables are dietary factors in the prevention of a number of cancers.

References

1. National Institutes of Health (Robert A. Gordon, editorial director). Cholesterol and noncardiovascular mortality. *J.A.M.A.* 244:25, 1980.

2. Garcia-Palmieri, M.R., Sorlie, P.D., Costas, R., Havlik, R.J. An apparent inverse relationship between serum cholesterol and cancer mortality in Puerto Rico. *Am. J. Epidemiol.* 114:29–40, 1981.

3. Williams, R.R., Sorlie, P.D., Feinleib, M., et al. Cancer incidence by levels of cholesterol. *J.A.M.A.* 245:247–252, 1981.

4. Kozarevic, D., McGee, D., Vojvodic, N., et al. Serum cholesterol and mortality: The Yugoslavia Cardiovascular Disease Study. *Am. J. Epidemiol.* 114:21–28, 1981.

5. Kessler, I., Clark, J.P. Saccharin, cyclamate, and human bladder cancer. *J.A.M.A.* 240:349–355, 1978.

6. Hoover, R. Artificial sweeteners and human bladder cancer. *Lancet* 1:837–840, 1980.

7. Howe, G.R., Burch, J.D., Miller, A.B., et al. Artificial sweeteners and human bladder cancer. *Lancet* 2:578–581, 1977.

8. Howe, G.R., Burch, J.D., Miller, A.B., et al. Tobacco use, occupation, coffee, various nutrients, and bladder cancer. *J. Natl. Cancer Inst.* 64:701–713, 1980.

9. Martinez, I. Factors associated with cancer of the esophagus, mouth, and pharynx, in Puerto Rico. *J. Natl. Cancer Inst.* 42:1069–1094, 1969.

10. Wynder, E.L., Bross, I.J. Aetiological factors in mouth cancer. *Br. Med. J.* 1:1137–1143, 1957.

11. Rothman, K., Keller, A. The effect of joint exposure to alcohol and tobacco on risk of cancer of the mouth and pharynx. *J. Chronic Dis.* 25:711–716, 1972.

12. Graham, S., Dayal, H., Rohrer, T., et al. Dentition, diet, tobacco, and alcohol in the epidemiology of oral cancer. *J. Natl. Cancer Inst.* 59:1611–1616, 1977.

13. Schwartz, D., Lellouch, J., Flamant, R., Denoix, P.F. Alcool et cancer: Résultats d'une enquête rétrospective. *Rev. Franc. Etudes Clin. Biol.* 7:590–604, 1962.

14. Higginson, J. Etiological factors in gastrointestinal cancer in man. *J. Natl. Cancer Inst.* 37:527–545, 1966.

15. Dawber, T.R., Pearson, G., Anderson, P., et al. Dietary assessment in the epidemiologic study of coronary heart disease: The Framingham Study. II. Reliability of measurement. *Am. J. Clin. Nutr.* 11:226–233, 1962.

16. Nomura, A., Hankin, J.H., Rhoads, G.G. The reproducibility of dietary intake data in a prospective study of gastrointestinal cancer. *Am. J. Clin. Nutr.* 29:1432–1436, 1976

17. Reshef, A., Epstein, L.M. Reliability of a dietary questionnaire. *Am. J. Clin. Nutr.* 25:91–95, 1972.

18. Marshall, J., Priore, R., Haughey, B., et al. Spouse-subject interviews and the reliability of diet studies. *Am. J. Epidemiol.* 112:675–683, 1980.

19. Kolonel, N., Hirohata, T., Nomura, A. Adequacy of survey data collection from substitute respondents. *Am. J. Epidemiol.* 106:476–484, 1977.

20. Bingham, S., McNeil, N., Cummings, J.H. The diet of individuals: A study of a randomly-chosen cross section of British adults in a Cambridgeshire village. *Br. J. Nutr.* 45:23–35, 1981.

21. Gersovitz, M., Madden, J.P., Smiciklas-Wright, H. Validity of the 24-hour dietary recall and seven-day record for group comparisons. *J. Am. Diet. Assoc.* 73:48–55, 1978.

22. Reddy, B.S., Wynder, E.L. Metabolic epidemiology of colon cancer: Fecal bile acids and neutral sterols in colon cancer patients and patients with adenomatous polyps. *Cancer* 39:2533–2539, 1977.

23. Reddy, B.S., Hedges, A., Laakso, K., Wynder, E.L. Fecal constituents of a high-risk North American and a low-risk Finnish population for the development of large bowel cancer. *Cancer Lett.* 4:217–222, 1978.

24. Aries, V.C., Crowther, J.S., Drasar, B.S., et al. The effect of a strict vegetarian diet on the faecal flora and faecal steroid concentration. *J. Pathol.* 103:54–56, 1971.

25. Cummings, J. Dietary fibre, transit-time, faecal bacteria, steroids, and colon cancer in two Scandinavian populations. *Lancet* 2:207–211, 1977.

26. Haenszel, W., Berg, J.W., Segi, M., et al. Large-bowel cancer in Hawaiian Japanese. *J. Natl. Cancer Inst.* 51:1765–1779, 1973.

27. Haenszel, W., Locke, F.B., Segi, M. A case-control study of large bowel cancer in Japan. *J. Natl. Cancer Inst.* 64:17–22, 1980.

28. Wynder, E.L. The epidemiology of large bowel cancer. *Cancer Res.* 35:3388–3394, 1975.

29. Graham, S., Dayal, H., Swanson, M., et al. Diet in the epidemiology of cancer of the colon and rectum. *J. Natl. Cancer Inst.* 61:709–714, 1978.

30. Bjelke, E. Epidemiologic studies of cancer of the stomach, colon and rectum, with special emphasis on the role of diet. Ph.D. dissertation, University of Minnesota. Ann Arbor: University Microfilms, 1973.

31. Graham, S., Mettlin, C. Diet and colon cancer. *Am. J. Epidemiol.* 109:1–20, 1979.

32. Eastwood, M.A., Kirkpatrick, J.R., Mitchell, W.D., et al. Effects of dietary supplements of wheat bran and cellulose on faeces and bowel function. *Br. Med. J.* 4:392–394, 1973.

33. Burkitt, D.P., Walker, A.R., Painter, N.S. Effect of dietary fibre on stools and transit-times, and its role in the causation of diseases. *Lancet* 2:1408–1412, 1972.

34. Fleiszer, D., Murray, D., MacFarlane, J., Brown, R.A. Protective effect of dietary fibre against chemically induced bowel tumors in rats. *Lancet* 1:552–553, 1978.

35. Ward, J.M., Yamanoto, R.S., Weisburger, J.H. Cellulose dietary bulk and azoxy-methane-induced intestinal cancer. *J. Natl. Cancer Inst.* 51:713–715, 1973.

36. Wilson, R.B., Hutcheson, D.P., Wideman, L. Dimethylhydrazine-induced colon tumors in rats fed diets containing beef fat or corn oil with and without wheat bran. *Am. J. Clin. Nutr.* 30:176–181, 1977.

37. Cruse, J.P., Lewin, M.R., Clark, C.G. Failure of bran to protect against experimental colon cancer in rats. *Lancet* 2:1278–1279, 1978.

38. Asp, N., Bauer, H., Dahlquist, A., et al. Dietary fibre and experimental colon cancer in the rat. *Nutr. Cancer* 1:70–73, 1979.

39. Burkitt, D.P., Walker, A.R.P., Painter, N.S. Effect of dietary fibre on stools and transit-times, and its role in the causation of diseases. *Lancet* 2:1408–1412, 1972.

40. Modan, B., Barell, V., Lubin, F., et al. Low-fiber intake as an etiologic factor in cancer of the colon. *J. Natl. Cancer Inst.* 55:15–18, 1975.

41. Dales, L.G., Friedman, G.D., Ury, H.K., et al. A case-control study of relationships of diet and other traits to colorectal cancer in blacks. *Am. J. Epidemiol.* 109:132–144, 1978.

42. Graham, S., Mettlin, C., Marshall, J. et al. Dietary factors in the epidemiology of cancer of the larynx. *Am. J. Epidemiol.* 113:675–680, 1981.

43. Saffiotti, U., Montesano, R., Sellakumar, A.R., Boorg, S.A. Experimental cancer of the lung. *Cancer* 20:857–864, 1964.

44. Chu, S.W., Malmgren, R.A. An inhibitory effect of vitamin A on the induction of tumors of the forestomach and cervix in the Syrian hamster by carcinogenic polycyclic hydrocarbons. *Cancer Res.* 25:884–895, 1965.

45. Nettesheim, P., Williams, M.L. The influence of vitamin A on the susceptibility of the rat lung to 3-methylcholanthrene. *Int. J. Cancer* 17:351–357, 1976.

46. Newberne, P.M., Suphakarn, V. Preventive role of vitamin A in colon carcinogenesis in rats. *Cancer* 40:2553–2556, 1977.

47. Merriman, R.L., Bertram, J.S. Reversible inhibition by retinoids of 3-methyl-cholanthrene-induced neoplastic transformation in C3H/10T1/2 clone 8 cells. *Cancer Res.* 39:1661–1666, 1979.

48. Hirayama, T. Diet and cancer. *Nutr. Cancer* 1:67–81, 1979.

49. Bjelke, E. Dietary vitamin A and human lung cancer. *Int. J. Cancer* 15:561–565, 1975.

50. MacLennan, R., Da Costa, J., Day, N.E., et al. Risk factors for lung cancer in Singapore Chinese: A population with high female incidence rates. *Int. J. Cancer* 20:854–860, 1977.

51. Kark, J.D., Smith, A.H., Switzer, B.R., Hames, C.G. Serum vitamin A (retinol) and cancer incidence in Evans County, Georgia. *J. Natl. Cancer Inst.* 66:7–16, 1981.

52. Mettlin, C., Graham, S., Swanson, M. Vitamin A and lung cancer. *J. Natl. Cancer Inst.* 62:1435–1438, 1979.

53. Mettlin, C., Graham, S. Dietary risk factors in human bladder cancer. *Am. J. Epidemiol.* 110:255–263, 1979.

54. Mettlin, C., Graham, S., Priore, R., et al. Diet and cancer of the esophagus. *Nutr. Cancer* 2:143–147, 1981.

55. Wattenberg, L.W., Loub, W.D. Inhibition of polycyclic aromatic hydrocarbon induced neoplasia by naturally occurring indoles. *Cancer Res.* 38:1410–1413, 1978.

56. Wattenberg, L.W. Effects of dietary constituents on the metabolism of chemical carcinogens. *Cancer Res.* 35:3326–3331, 1975.

7 Nutritional Care of Hospitalized Patients

Eleanor A. Young, Ph.D.

Medicine and clinical nutrition interface in a vibrant, interrelated, and dynamic manner [1–6] (Figure 7-1). This interface occurs at the cellular level of biochemical reactions, at the organ and total body levels where physiologic responses are dependent on essential nutrients, at the psychological and behavioral levels of human behavior, and at the deepest levels of the human spirit. Moreover, medicine and nutrition interface not only with each other, but also with the science, technology, and art of delivering health care [1]. Sensitive, complex, and dynamic human values of the patient, his or her family and friends, and the personnel involved in the health care delivery system are important considerations of this interface between medicine and clinical nutrition.

Factors Involved in the Nutritional Care of Hospitalized Patients: Advances and Limitations

Many factors have contributed to our present understanding of the nutritional needs of hospitalized patients, and have thus provided significant advances in the science and technology of providing nutritional support.

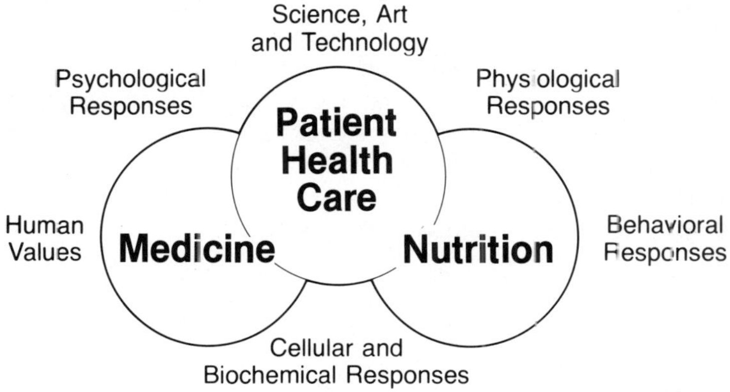

Figure 7-1. Factors that interact in the nutritional care of hospitalized patients.

Table 7-1
Nutritional Care of Hospitalized Patients: Advances and Limitations

1. Greater public awareness of the role of nutrition in health and disease
2. Emphasis on nutrition education for physicians and health care professionals
3. Reports of iatrogenic malnutrition in hospital patients
4. Advances in technical support systems
5. Development and refinement of approaches to nutritional assessment
6. Advances in our understanding of the nutritional needs of hospitalized patients
7. Development of approaches to provide nutritional support
   a. Natural foods ingested orally
   b. Therapeutic diets
   c. Special supplements
   d. Defined formula diets for oral or enteral alimentation
   e. Parenteral nutrition
      (1) Central venous
      (2) Peripheral

Some of these factors are given in Table 7-1. It is difficult to quantitate the specific contributions of each of these factors, yet it is clear that each one has made unique contributions over the past decade or two. There are also limitations to our understanding of nutritional care of hospitalized patients; these limitations serve to provide directions for future study.

Greater Public Awareness of the Role of Nutrition in Health and Disease

Everywhere one looks, nutrition seems to be a focus of consideration in various media: radio, television, books and magazine articles, and even casual conversation [7–12]. Thus the hospitalized patient and his or her family are more attuned to nutrition and more sophisticated in asking questions and seeking information concerning nutritional status. In many cases the patient is more capable of entering into his or her own nutritional therapy, and does so with greater knowledge of nutrition facts, although in some instances also with considerable nutrition misinformation [11,12].

Emphasis on Nutrition Education for Physicians and Other Health Care Professionals

It has been recognized that there is inadequate coverage of nutrition in the curriculum of most medical schools in the United States [13–16], and a concerted effort has been put forth to provide greater emphasis on nutrition education for physicians and other health care professionals [17–19], as evidenced by the development and funding of thirteen interdisciplinary nutrition curriculum development programs and seven clinical nutrition research units. This kind of emphasis on nutrition education for physicians and other health care professionals is clearly a positive step toward providing more comprehensive nutritional support for hospitalized patients. A number of training programs that have been designed to enhance nutrition education have been interdisciplinary in nature. The involvement of physicians, nurses, nutritionists, pharmacists, and other health care personnel in the nutritional care of hospitalized patients has broadened the scope of awareness of nutritional care and has strengthened the delivery system to provide this care.

Reports of Iatrogenic Malnutrition in Hospitalized Patients

The reports of malnutrition in hospitalized patients [20–37] have focused attention on the need to provide nutritional support for this population group (Table 7-2). Moreover, most of these reports have documented iatrogenic malnutrition, that is, a worsening of nutritional status during hospitalization resulting from negligence in providing adequate nutritional support under conditions when it could and should have been provided. In 1965 Leevy and colleagues [20] were among the first to report deficient nutrient intake (39%) and hypovitaminemia (59%) in 120 randomly selected patients surveyed in a large municipal hospital. It was Butterworth [22,23] who brought nationwide attention to the "skeleton in the hospital closet," clearly documenting iatrogenic malnutrition in hospitalized patients. Since that time, there have continued to be reports of the prevalence of malnutrition in U.S. hospitals [24–37]. Some of the factors contributing to hospital malnutrition have been identified (Table 7-3).

Advances in Technical Support Systems

Advances in technical support systems have provided considerable improvement in the nutritional support of hospitalized patients. Processing of nutritional formulas and supplements and the manufacturing of new types of equipment such as delivery pumps and catheters have enabled a more sophisticated, efficient nutrient delivery system to be utilized.

Development and Refinement of Approaches to Nutritional Assessment

The development and refinement of new approaches to nutritional assessment have also contributed in a major way to providing nutritional support for hospitalized patients [38–42]. Many hospital centers around the country

Table 7–2
Malnutrition in Hospitalized Patients

Authors	*Date*	*Type of Patient and Hospital*	*Percentage of Patients with Malnutrition*
Leevy et al. [20]	1965	Randomly selected Municipal hospital	39–59
Bollet and Owens [21]	1973	Medical/surgical Municipal hospital	17–45
Butterworth [22]	1974	Medical/surgical Municipal teaching hospital	23–56
Butterworth [23]	1974	Surgical Municipal teaching hospital	27–53
Bistrian et al. [24]	1974	Surgical Municipal teaching hospital	12–80
Trubowitz et al. [25]	1974	Medical V.A. hospital	10–15
Blackburn and Bistrian [26]	1974	Surgical Municipal teaching hospital	1–79 (mean: 50)
Bistrian et al. [27]	1976	General medical Municipal teaching hospital	44–76
Tobias and Van Itallie [28]	1977	General medical Municipal teaching hospital	91[a]
Weinsier et al. [29]	1979	General medical Municipal teaching hospital	48 (on admission) 69 (follow-up)
Tomaiolo and Kraus [30]	1980	Nonindigent alcoholics	36
Willard et al. [31]	1980	Medical/surgical Private community hospital	31.5
Bansal et al. [32]	1980	Unselected dialysis patients	19
Lemoine et al. [33]	1980	Medical General hospital	11–33 (mean: 30)
Parsons et al. [34]	1980	Medical/surgical Pediatric teaching hospital	12–30
Driver and LeBrun [35]	1980	Medical, ventilatory support patients V.A. center	36–71
Kien and Camitta [36]	1981	Pediatric cancer patients Municipal medical center	20–48
Pollack et al. [37]	1982	Pediatric ICU Municipal medical center	37

[a]Actual or potential malnutrition.

have developed an interdisciplinary team approach to nutritional care [43–47]. This provides a broad base of expertise that is applied to the nutritional needs of the patient. Recent approaches to nutritional assessment utilize modern computer technology, programmed calculators, nomograms,

Table 7-3
Factors Contributing to Malnutrition in Hospitalized Patients

1. Height and weight not recorded
2. Frequent rotation of staff
3. Use of glucose and saline infusions for prolonged periods
4. Diffusion of patient care responsibilities
5. Withholding meals for diagnostic tests
6. Food intake of patients not monitored
7. Inadequate and inappropriate tube feedings
8. Lack of knowledge of vitamin preparations and other supplements
9. Failure to recognize increased nutritional needs as a result of injury or disease
10. Inadequate nutritional preparation of patients prior to surgery
11. Lack of nutritional support in the prevention of and recovery from infection
12. Delay of nutritional support until the patient is in an advanced state of depletion
13. Inadequate communication between physician and other professional personnel
14. Laboratory tests for nutritional assessment
    a. Limited availability
    b. Inappropriate use
    c. Failure to use

Source: Adapted from Butterworth [22,23].

and automated hospital information systems for compiling and assessing nutrition data [48–53].

While many advances have been made in nutritional assessment, there are still a number of major limitations in the practical application of assessment methods [54]. Unfortunately, there is no single measurement that is a satisfactory measure of nutritional status. Although skinfold measurements may reflect body fat stores, and mid-arm muscle circumference may reflect lean body mass, wide individual differences in such measurements make interpretation difficult [55,56]. Delayed cutaneous hypersensitivity to antigens may occur not only in malnutrition but also in fever, tumors, shock, sepsis, and steroid therapy, and thus is not specific only for nutritional status [57]. Serum albumin and transferrin levels reflect severe protein-calorie malnutrition but are not sensitive enough measures to assess subclinical malnutrition [42,58]. It has been suggested that plasma thyroxine-binding prealbumin and retinol-binding protein may be more sensitive measures [58–60]; however, the former may be modulated by iron status, energy restriction, and renal disease, while the latter may be influenced by infection, vitamin A deficiency, thyroid status, liver disease, and zinc deficiency [58]. The search for more specific methods to determine nutritional status is growing in intensity. Controlled studies are needed to determine the effectiveness of newly proposed methods. Repeated assessment and longitudinal assessment studies are needed to test the reliability and validity of methods, and the changes that may occur with time. We need to search for appropriate combinations of anthropometric, biochemical, and functional techniques that may be useful in nutritional assessment. We also need to determine standards and criteria for nutritional assessment for specific age groups, such as infants, adolescents, and the elderly, and for specific disease states.

Advances in Understanding the Nutritional Needs of Hospitalized Patients

Advances in our knowledge and understanding of the nutritional needs of hospitalized patients are of utmost importance. Our present knowledge with respect to modification of the nutritional needs of patients with specific disorders or diseases is very limited. As shown in Table 7-4, recent efforts have been made to assess these needs for specific groups of patients [61–72]. Nutritional assessment of these patients takes on special characteristics based on unique physical, physiologic, or metabolic features of the particular problems or conditions of the patient. We need to learn a great deal more about the requirements for and metabolism of specific nutrients in patients with different disorders or disease states.

While attention has been directed to the energy and protein requirements of patients following severe burns [73–76], relatively few studies have been concerned with fuel metabolism under other conditions or disease states. Warnold and colleagues [77] have sought to define the upper and lower range of energy needs that can be expected in hospital patients, and thereby to define patients at risk for energy needs. It has been pointed out by Freinkel [78] that the prevailing needs of clinical medicine demand important contributions from nutrition science. These contributions include (1) the dose-response relationships and duration of hormonal action in response to dietary manipulations; (2) the regulatory impact of substrate interaction, that is, how the metabolism of one fuel affects that of another; (3) modification of fuel metabolism via disparate effects in selected organs; and (4) possible modula-

Table 7–4
Nutritional Assessment of Patients with Special Problems

1. Energy requirements for patients on respirators
2. Protein losses in peritoneal dialysis
3. Nutritional needs and immune responses in neoplastic disease
4. Malnutrition and nutritional support in hepatic failure
5. Vitamin deficiencies in dialysis patients
6. Nutritional needs of the patient with spinal cord injury
7. Nutritional assessment of patients with head or neck cancer
8. Nutritional needs of neonatal and pediatric patients
9. Nutritional support for critically ill patients with severe stress, trauma burns

tions by the central nervous system in maintaining homeostasis of metabolic fuels [78].

Provision of Nutritional Support for Hospitalized Patients

Finally, in providing nutritional support to hospitalized patients, attention must be focused on the method of alimentation that is most appropriate for each patient. Possibilities for feeding include natural foods ingested orally, therapeutic diets, special nutritional supplements, defined formula diets for oral or enteral alimentation, and parenteral alimentation delivered by the central venous or vein route.

Under normal circumstances, oral feeding of natural foods is the optimal method of supplying energy and essential nutrients. Palatability, acceptability, and the lower cost of natural foods make this the method of choice if the patient has an adequate functioning intestine, is capable of eating, and does not have any physical, physiologic, or metabolic reasons to preclude the intake of natural foods. With modern blenders it is possible to liquefy almost all foods so that they can be consumed in a liquid form if this is necessary.

Modification in the quality, quantity, or pattern of food intake is necessary for a variety of therapeutic diets. Most hospitals have available a manual of therapeutic diets, and these diets should be orderd by physicians according to the needs of the patient. A number of therapeutic diets are not only effective for nutritional management, but they constitute the most important modality in the medical management of the patient. Examples of therapeutic diets that may be effective include a gluten-free diet in gluten enteropathy, lactose restriction in lactose malabsorption, lipid restriction in hyperlipidemias, protein restriction in renal failure and in hepatic disease with encephalopathy, energy restriction in obesity, selective restriction of amino acids in specific inborn error of metabolism, and modification of dietary carbohydrate and fat in patients with insulin-dependent diabetes. To ensure the efficacy of these therapeutic diets and compliance by the patient, the patient must understand that the diet is an important aspect of overall medical management. The rationale of the diet should be carefully explained to the patient, and dietary counseling should be provided when this is appropriate. It is likewise necessary for the patient to have a clear concept of the appropriate time frame for application of the diet—for example, is the diet necessary throughout life (gluten restriction in celiac sprue, galactose restriction in galactosemia), or is the diet a temporary measure pending the achievement of a defined goal? Without these considerations given to the prescription of a therapeutic diet, the likelihood of compliance, and therefore of the efficacy of the diet, is likely to be minimal. For example, West [79,80] has extensively explored reasons for noncompliance in the diabetic diet and has found contributing factors to include the considerations just discussed.

Table 7–5
Contraindications to Oral Feeding

1. Mechanical difficulties in chewing
2. Impairment of swallowing mechanisms
3. Coma
4. Gastrointestinal obstruction
5. Fistulas of the upper gastrointestinal tract
6. Severe vomiting
7. Severe and persistent anorexia
8. Symptomatic exacerbation of disease with oral intake
9. Severe malabsorption/diarrhea exacerbated by oral intake

Table 7–6
Considerations for Alternative Feeding

1. Nutritional/medical status of the patient
2. Safety and potential risks involved
3. Acceptance of alternative feeding method by the patient/family
4. Medical capacity to offer alternative nutritional support
5. Cost-benefit ratio to the patient and to the hospital

Although oral feeding of natural foods is preferable, alternative methods of feeding may be essential for patients when there are contraindications to oral feeding (Table 7-5). When alternate feeding becomes a viable option for nutritional support, a number of considerations become important in selecting the most effective method (Table 7-6).

Tube feeding is an option for nutritional support when an adequate absorbing surface is available in the gastrointestinal tract. The enteral route is a first consideration of alternate feeding because it is simple, economical, and well tolerated by most patients compared to parenteral alimentation. In addition, luminal nutrition is necessary to maintain the structural and functional integrity of the small intestines [81]. Within the past decade, there has been an ever-expanding variety of specific clinical conditions in which enteral feeding merits consideration [81–87]. Some indications for enteral feedings are given in Table 7-7. The selection of the feeding formula and the route of administration are important considerations. A wide variety of formulas are currently available [82–87], and careful consideration should be given to making the most effective choice. In general, these formulas fall under three categories: monomeric, polymeric, and modular [82–85]. The nutritive composition of these diets varies widely, thus complicating the choice. Some formulas are designed to provide all essential nutrients, while others are designed to supplement other nutritional support, such as simultaneous jejunostomy

Table 7–7
Indications for Enteral Feeding

1. Gastrointestinal disease
   - Inflammatory bowel disease
   - Pancreatitis
   - Fistulas
   - Malabsorption syndromes
   - Short-bowel syndrome
2. Cancer
3. Anorexia
4. Acute renal failure
5. Cardiac disease
6. Hypermetabolic states: trauma, infection, burns
7. Inborn errors of metabolism

Table 7–8
Complications of Enteral Feeding

Nonmetabolic	*Metabolic*
Aspiration	Hyperglycemia, glucosuria
Vomiting	Electrolyte imbalance
Diarrhea, abdominal cramping	Hyperosmolar coma
Esophageal erosion	Edema
Vitamin deficiency	
Essential fatty acid deficiency	
Clogging of tube lumen	

feeding and peripheral vein nutrition. There are also a number of possible routes of administration: oral, nasoenteral, esophagostomy, gastrostomy, and jejunostomy. Continuous-drip infusion of enteral formulas has been found to be the easiest, safest, and best tolerated method of administration. Patients must be monitored closely so as to avoid or minimize complications [82–87]. The most frequently reported complications of enteral tube feeding are given in Table 7-8.

The application of enteral feeding for hospital patients has been extensive over the past decade; however, carefully controlled clinical trials as well as basic animal studies are needed to substantiate the efficacy and cost-effectiveness ratio of this approach to nutritional support [82,86,88–90]. Many questions regarding the uses of these defined formula diets remain to be answered (Table 7-9).

When enteral nutrition is contraindicated or inadequate to meet the essential nutritional needs of the patient, parenteral nutrition becomes the

Table 7–9
Needs and Future Considerations for Enteral Nutrition Support

1. Carefully designed and implemented clinical trials to document efficiency in various disease states
2. Assessment of the effect of nutrient variations on digestion and absorption of nutrients
3. Assessment of the effect of the route of administration on digestion and absorption of nutrients
4. Influence of enteral formulas on:
   gastric emptying
   gut microflora
   liver lipid
   pancreatic enzyme responses
   intestinal enzyme responses
   biliary responses
   hormonal responses

only remaining alternative to nutritional support. Over the past decade and a half, there has been extensive clinical experience with total parenteral nutrition (TPN) [91–94]. A great deal has been learned regarding the formulation, administration, and complications of TPN, as well as the patient's metabolic response. This approach to nutritional support requires expertise in preparation of the formulas, in maintaining a sterile and safe environment, and in monitoring the patient. It has been well documented that TPN is lifesaving in a variety of clinical situations, including obstructing lesions of the gastrointestinal tract, fistulas, acute inflammatory bowel disease, severe malabsorptive states, hypermetabolic states (burns, trauma, sepsis), congenital anomalies in the neonate prior to surgery, and prolonged coma.

In recent years, attention has been focused on the metabolism of body fuels [95–97] and body composition [98] during TPN, the nutritional adequacy of formulas [91,99–101], the nutritional status of patients receiving TPN [102–109], the efficacy of TPN in various clinical circumstances [92–94,97,98,102,110–113], prolonged home TPN [114–117], and alternate carbohydrate sources for TPN [118–119].

Peripheral-vein amino acid therapy has been shown to result in maintaining nitrogen balance, preserving the lean body mass while blood glucose levels are maintained and fatty acids are released from the adipose stores [94,120–122]. Indications for use of this therapy require further evaluation. Peripheral parenteral infusion with lipid has been shown to be effective in adding caloric intake as well as providing a source of essential fatty acids [123–124].

Clinical judgment is needed in deciding on the most appropriate method of supplying the essential nutrients. The nondepleted postoperative patient requiring nutritional support may do well on peripheral nutrition or on continuous jejunal feeding. The depleted postoperative patient, whose caloric and protein needs are higher than that of the nondepleted patient, may require continuous enteral feeding plus peripheral nutrition. On the other hand, the hypermetabolic, hypercatabolic patient may require total nutritional support via central venous line. Caution is needed to avoid the complications of excessive total formula and/or carbohydrate infusion [122, 125–129].

Summary

Medicine and clinical nutrition interface in a dynamic manner that must also take into consideration the complex human values of the patient and of the personnel of the health care delivery system. Technological advances, public awareness of the role of nutrition in health and disease, and increasing emphasis on nutrition education for medical personnel have made it possible to provide good and appropriate nutritional support for hospitalized patients.

Recognition of the existence of iatrogenic malnutrition in hospitalized patients has focused attention on identifying the responsible factors. Yet limitations in accurate nutritional assessment and understanding of nutritional needs of patients with specific disorders have hampered success in improving the dietary regimens of hospitalized patients. While the optimal nutritional support is obtained by natural foods taken by mouth, technological advances have made it possible to satisfy a broad variety of therapeutic dietary needs. Considerations for the most appropriate choice of nutritional supports have been discussed.

References

1. Blackburn, G.L. Interaction of the science of nutrition and the science of medicine. *J.P.E.N.* 3:131–136, 1979.

2. Olson, R.E. Clinical nutrition, an interface between human ecology and internal medicine. *Nutr. Rev.* 36:161–178, 1978.

3. Lowenberg, M.E., Todhunter, E.N., Wilson, E.D., et al. *Food and Man*. New York: John Wiley and Sons, 1974. P. 163.

4. Young, E.A. Nutrition—An essential aspect of the medical curriculum. In *Nutrition Education in Medical Schools*. Hearing before the Subcom-

mittee on Nutrition of the Committee on Agriculture, Nutrition and Forestry, U.S. Senate, 95th Congress, September 20, 1978. Washington, D.C.: Government Printing Office, 1978. Pp. 60–85.

5. Young, E.A. Nutrition—An essential component of health and of health care. *J. Am. Coll. Nutr.* 1:227–237, 1982.

6. Darby, W.J. The renaissance of nutrition education. *Nutr. Rev.* 35:33–38, 1977.

7. Olson, J.C., and Sims, L.S. Assessing nutrition knowledge from an information processing perspective. *J. Nutr. Ed.* 12:157–160, 1980.

8. United States Food and Drug Administration. *Food and Nutrition: Knowledge and Beliefs. A Nationwide Study Among Food Shoppers.* Princeton, N.J.: Response Analysis, 1974.

9. Walker, M.A., Hill, M.M. *Homemakers' Food and Nutrition Knowledge, Practices and Opinions.* United States Department of Agriculture, Home Economics Research Report no. 39. Washington, D.C.: Government Printing Office, 1975.

10. Jacoby, J., Chestnut, R.W., Silberman, W. Consumer use and comprehension of nutritional information. *J. Consumer Res.* 4:119–128, 1977.

11. Herbert, V., and Barrett, S. *Vitamins and Health Foods: The Great American Hustle.* Philadelphia: George F. Stickley, 1981.

12. Editors of Consumer Reports Books. *Health Quackery.* New York: Holt, Rinehart and Winston, 1980.

13. Cyborski, C. Nutrition content in medical curriculum. *J. Nutr. Ed.* 9:17–18, 1977.

14. American Medical Association. Current status of nutrition in medical curricula: Changes since the 1976 survey. In *Nutrition Education in Medical Schools.* Hearings before the Subcommittee on Nutrition and the Committee on Agriculture, Nutrition and Forestry, U.S. Senate. Washington, D.C.: Government Printing Office, 1978. Pp. 107–111.

15. *Nutrition Education in Medical Schools.* Hearings before the Subcommittee on Nutrition of the Committee on Agriculture, Nutrition and Forestry, U.S. Senate, September 20, 1978. Washington, D.C.: Government Printing Office, 1978.

16. Division of Medicine, Bureau of Health Manpower, Health Resources Administration and the Nutrition Foundation, Inc. Evaluation of nutrition curriculum at nine selected medical schools. In *Hearings on Diet Related to Killer Disease, VIII.* U.S. Senate, Select Committee on Nutrition and Human Needs. Washington, D.C.: Government Printing Office, 1978. Pp. 65–79.

17. Joint Committee on Human Nutrition Research of the Committee on Health and Medicine and the Committee on Food and Renewable Resources, Federal Coordinating Council on Science, Engineering and Technology, Office of Science and Technology Policy, Executive Office of the

President. *Federally-Supported Human Nutrition Research, Training and Education: Update for the 1980s. I. Human Nutrition Research and Training. Am. J. Clin. Nutr.* 34:978–1030, 1981.

18. Fredrickson, D.S. Federally supported human nutrition research, training and education. *Am. J. Clin. Nutr.* 34:957–958, 1981.

19. Olson, R.E. Clinical nutrition in the hospital setting: An American perspective. *Recent Adv. Clin. Nutr.* 1:287–292, 1981.

20. Leevy, C.M., Cardi, L., Frank, O., et al. Incidence and significance of hypovitaminemia in a randomly selected municipal hospital population. *Am. J. Clin. Nutr.* 17:259–271, 1965.

21. Bollet, A.J., Owens, S. Evaluation of nutritional status of selected hospitalized patients. *Am. J. Clin. Nutr.* 26:931–938, 1973.

22. Butterworth, C.E. The skeleton in the hospital closet. *Nutrition Today* 9:4–8, 1974.

23. Butterworth, C.E. Malnutrition in the hospital. *J.A.M.A.* 230:879, 1974.

24. Bistrian, B.R., Blackburn, G.L., Hallowell, E., Heddle, R. Protein status of general surgical patients. *J.A.M.A.* 230:858–860, 1974.

25. Trubowitz, S., Frank, O., Baker, H. Survey of vitamin B_{12} and folate in the serum and marrow tissue of hospitalized patients. *Am. J. Clin. Nutr.* 27:580–583, 1974.

26. Blackburn, G.L., Bistrian, B. A report from Boston. *Nutrition Today* 10:30, 1974.

27. Bistrian, B.R., Blackburn, G.L., Vitale, J., et al. Prevalence of malnutrition in general medical patients. *J.A.M.A.* 235:1567–1570, 1976.

28. Tobias, A.L., Van Itallie, T.B. Nutritional problems of hospitalized patients. *J. Am. Diet. Assoc.* 71:253–256, 1977.

29. Weinsier, R.L., Hunker, E.M., Krumdieck, C.L., Butterworth, C.E. Hospital malnutrition. A prospective evaluation of general medical patients during the course of hospitalization. *Am. J. Clin. Nutr.* 32:418–426, 1979.

30. Tomaiolo, P.P., Kraus, V. Nutritional status of hospitalized alcoholic patients. *J.P.E.N.* 4:1–3, 1980.

31. Willard, M.D., Giladorf, R.B., Price, R.A. Protein-calorie malnutrition in a community hospital. *J.A.M.A.* 243:1720–1722, 1980.

32. Bansal, V.K., Popli, S., Pickering, J., et al. Protein-calorie malnutrition and cutaneous energy in hemodialysis maintained patients. *Am. J. Clin. Nutr.* 33:1608–1611, 1980.

33. Lemoine, A., Le Devehat, C., Codaccioni, J.L., et al. Vitamin B_1, B_2, B_6 and C status in hospital inpatients. *Am. J. Clin. Nutr.* 33:2595–2600, 1980.

34. Parsons, H.G., Francoeur, T.E., Howland, P., et al. The nutritional status of hospitalized children. *Am. J. Clin. Nutr.* 33:1140–1146, 1980.

35. Driver, A.G., LeBrun, M. Iatrogenic malnutrition in patients receiving ventilatory support. *J.A.M.A.* 244:2195–2196, 1980.

36. Kien, C.L., Camitta, B.M. Protein-energy nutritional status of pediatric cancer. *Am. J. Clin. Nutr.* 34:2486–2492, 1981.

37. Pollack, M.M., Wiley, J.S., Kanter, R., Holbrook, P.R. Malnutrition in critically ill infants and children. *J.P.E.N.* 6:20–24, 1982.

38. Wilmore, D.W. *The Metabolic Management of the Critically Ill.* New York: Plenum Medical Book Co., 1977.

39. Weinsier, R.L., Butterworth, C.E., Jr. *Handbook of Clinical Nutrition.* St. Louis: C.V. Mosby, 1981.

40. Blackburn, G.L., Bistrian, B.R., Maini, B.S., et al. *Manual for Nutritional/Metabolic Assessment of the Hospitalized Patient.* Proceedings of the 62nd Annual Clinical Congress of the American College of Surgeons, Chicago, October 11–15, 1976. Boston: Nutrition Support Service, New England Deaconess Hospital, 1976.

41. Christakis, G. How to make a nutritional diagnosis: A. Adult nutritional diagnosis. In Barness, L.A., Coble, Y.D., MacDonald, D.I., Christakis, G. (Eds.), *Nutrition and Medical Practice.* Westport, Conn.: AVI Publishing Company, 1981. Pp. 3–17.

42. Michel, L., Serrano, A., Malt, R.A. Nutritional support of hospitalized patients. *N. Engl. J. Med.* 304:1147–1152, 1981.

43. Nehme, A.E. Nutritional support of the hospitalized patient. The team concept. *J.A.M.A.* 243:1906–1908, 1980.

44. Smith, A.E. Development of a coordinated total nutrition support service in a pediatric patient population. *Nutr. Supp. Serv.* 1:18–20, 1981.

45. Curtin, H.C., Harvey, R.F., Jellinek, H.M. Role of the clinical nutritionist as a member of a rehabilitation team. *Nutr. Supp. Serv.* 2:25–31, 1982.

46. Hopkins, R.J. Expanding the pharmacist's role in nutritional support service. *Nutr. Supp. Serv.* 1:20–23, 1981.

47. Medical Directions, Inc. *Establishing a Nutritional Support Service.* Chicago: Abbott Laboratories, 1980.

48. Danford, D.E. Computer applications to medical nutrition problems. *J.P.E.N.* 5:441–446, 1981.

49. Rich, A.J. A programable calculator system for the estimation of nutritional intake of hospital patients. *Am. J. Clin. Nutr.* 34:2276–2279, 1981.

50. Hoover, L.W., Leonard, M.S. Automated hospital information system functions for dietetics. *J. Am. Diet. Assoc.* 80:312–316, 1982.

51. Wright, P.D., Shearing, G., Rich, A.I., Johnston, I.D.A. The role of a computer in the management of clinical parenteral nutrition. *J.P.E.N.* 2:652–657, 1978.

52. Geller, R.J., Blackburn, S.A., Glendon, D.H., et al. Computer optimization of enteral hyperalimentation. *J.P.E.N.* 3:79–83, 1979.

53. Rainey-MacDonald, C.G., Holliday, R.L., Wells, G.A. Nomograms for predicting resting energy expenditure of hospitalized patients. *J.P.E.N.* 6:59–60, 1982.

54. Jeejeebhoy, K.N., Baker, J.P., Wolman, S.L., et al. Critical evaluation of the role of clinical assessment and body composition studies in patients with malnutrition and after total parenteral nutrition. *Am. J. Clin. Nutr.* 35:1117–1127, 1982.

55. Forse, R.A., Shizgal, H.M. The assessment of malnutrition. *Surgery* 88:17–24, 1980.

56. Fischer, J.E. Nutritional assessment before surgery. *Am. J. Clin. Nutr.* 35:1128–1131, 1982.

57. Cunningham-Rundles, S. Effects of nutritional status on immunological function. *Am. J. Clin. Nutr.* 35:1202–1210, 1982.

58. Golden, M.H.N. Transport proteins as indices of protein status. *Am. J. Clin. Nutr.* 35:1159–1165, 1982.

59. Shetty, P.S., Watrasiewicz, K.E., Jung, R.T., James, W.P.T. Rapid-turnover transport proteins: An index of subclinical protein energy malnutrition. *Lancet* 2:230–232, 1979.

60. Ingenbleek, Y., Shrieck, V.D., DeNayer, D., DeVisscher, M. The role of retinol-binding proteins in protein-calorie malnutrition. *Metabolism* 24:633–641, 1975.

61. McCamish, M.A., Dean, R.E., Quellette, T.R. Assessing energy requirements of patients on respirators. *J.P.E.N.* 5:513–516, 1981.

62. Mirtallo, J.M., Johnson, J.A., Fabri, P.J., Ruberg, R.L. Protein losses in peritoneal dialysis: A dilemma in nutritional support. *Nutr. Supp. Serv.* 2:14–17, 1982.

63. Kaminski, M.V., Nasr, N.J., Moss, A.J., et al. Nutritional status, immunity and survival in neoplastic disease. *Nutr. Supp. Serv.* 2:7–13, 1982.

64. Querica, R.A. Malnutrition and nutritional support in hepatic failure. *Nutr. Supp. Serv.* 1:22–24, 1981.

65. Cossa, J.P. Nutritional support of the patient in hepatic failure. *Nutr. Supp. Serv.* 1:39–40, 1981.

66. Partridge, J.C., Payne, M.L., Leisgang, J.J., et al. Water intoxication secondary to feeding mismanagement. *Am. J. Dis. Child.* 135:38–41, 1981.

67. Kleiner, M.J., Tate, S.S., Sullivan, J.F., Chami, J. Vitamin B_6 deficiency in maintenance dialysis patients: Metabolic effects of repletion. *Am. J. Clin. Nutr.* 33:1612–1619, 1980.

68. Juan, D., Elrazak, M.A. Hypophosphatemia in hospitalized patients. *J.A.M.A.* 242:163–164, 1979.

69. Warnold, I., Falkheden, T., Hulten, B., Isaksson, B. Energy intake and expenditure in selected groups of hospital patients. *Am. J. Clin. Nutr.* 31:742–749, 1978.

70. Peiffer, S.C., Blust, P., Leyson, J.F.J. Nutritional assessment of the spinal cord injured patient. *J. Am. Diet. Assoc.* 78:501–505, 1981.

71. Lambert, M.J., III. Nutritional assessment of the head and neck cancer patient. *Otolaryngol. Head Neck Surg.* 88:695–699, 1980.

72. Merritt, R.J., Suskind, R.M. Nutritional survey of hospitalized pediatric patients. *Am. J. Clin. Nutr.* 32:1320–1325, 1979.

73. Wilmore, D.W. Nutrition and metabolism following thermal injury. *Clin. Plast. Surg.* 1(4):603–619, 1974.

74. Wilmore, D.W., Moylan, J.A., Bristow, B.F., et al. Anabolic effects of human growth hormone and high calorie feedings following thermal injury. *Surg. Gynecol. Obstet.* 138:875–884, 1974.

75. Kien, C.L., Young, V.R., Rohrbaugh, D.K., Burke, J.F. Increased rates of whole body protein synthesis and breakdown in children recovering from burns. *Ann. Surg.* 187:383–391, 1978.

76. Curreri, P.W., Richmond, D., Marvin, J., Baxter, C.R. Dietary requirements of patients with major burns. *J. Am. Diet. Assoc.* 65:415–417, 1974.

77. Warnold, I., Falkheden, T., Hulten, B., Isaksson, B. Energy intake and expenditure in selected groups of hospital patients. *Am. J. Clin. Nutr.* 31:742–749, 1978.

78. Freinkel, N. The role of nutrition in medicine. *J.A.M.A.* 239:1868–1872, 1978.

79. West, K.M. Diet and diabetes. *Postgrad. Med.* 60:209–216, 1976.

80. West, K.M. Diet therapy of diabetes: An analysis of failure. *Ann. Intern. Med.* 79:425–434, 1973.

81. Levine, G.M. Role of oral intake in maintenance of gut mass and disaccharidase activity. *Gastroenterology* 67:975–982, 1974.

82. Heymsfield, S.B., Horowitz, J., Lawson, D.H. Enteral hyperalimentation. In Burke, E. (Ed.), *Developments in Digestive Diseases*, vol. 3. Philadelphia: Lea and Febiger, 1980. Pp. 59–83.

83. Heymsfield, S.B., Bethel, R.A., Ansley, J.D. Enteral hyperalimentation: An alternate to central venous hyperalimentation. *Ann. Intern. Med.* 90:63–71, 1979.

84. Shils, M.E. Enteral nutrition by tube. *Cancer Res.* 37:2432–2439, 1977.

85. Floch, M.H. *Nutrition and Diet Therapy in Gastrointestinal Disease.* New York: Plenum Medical Book Co., 1981. Pp. 327–344.

86. Koretz, R.L., Meyer, J.H. Elemental diets—facts and fantasies. *Gastroenterology* 78:393–410, 1980.

87. Shils, M.E., Randall, H.T. Diet and nutrition in the care of the surgical patient. In Goodhart, R.S., Shils, M.E. (Eds.), *Modern Nutrition in*

Health and Disease. Philadelphia: Lea and Febiger, 1981. Pp. 1082–1124.

88. Young, E.A., Cioletti, L.A., Winborn, W.B., et al. Comparative study of nutritional adaptation to defined formula diets in rats. *Am. J. Clin. Nutr.* 33:2106–2118, 1980.

89. Young, E.A., Cioletti, L.A., Traylor, J.B., Balderas, V. Gastrointestinal response to nutrient variation of defined formula diets. *J.P.E.N.* 5:478–484, 1981.

90. Young, E.A., Cioletti, L.A., Traylor, J.B., Balderas, V. Gastrointestinal response to oral versus gastric feeding of defined formula diets. *Am. J. Clin. Nutr.* 35:715–726, 1982.

91. Shils, M.E. Guidelines for total parenteral nutrition. *J.A.M.A.* 220:1721–1730, 1972.

92. Shils, M.E. Parenteral nutrition. In Goodhart, R.S., Shils, M.E. (Eds.), *Modern Nutrition in Health and Disease*. Philadelphia: Lea and Febiger, 1980. Pp. 1125–1152.

93. Fischer, J.E. Hyperalimentation. *Med. Clin. North Am.* 63:973–983, 1979.

94. Floch, M.H. *Nutrition and Diet Therapy in Gastrointestinal Disease.* New York: Plenum Medical Book Co., 1981. Pp. 345–358.

95. Long, J.M., III, Wilmore, D.W., Mason, A.D., Pruitt, B.A. Effect of carbohydrate and fat intake on nitrogen excretion during total intravenous feeding. *Ann. Surg.* 185:417–422, 1977.

96. Long, C.L., Crosby, B.A., Geiger, B.A., Kinney, J.M. Parenteral nutrition in the septic patient: Nitrogen balance, limiting plasma amino acids, and calorie to nitrogen ratios. *Am. J. Clin. Nutr.* 29:380–391, 1976.

97. Anderson, G.H., Patel, D.G., Jeejeebhoy, K.N. Design and evaluation by nitrogen balance and blood aminograms of an amino acid mixture for total parenteral nutrition of adults with gastrointestinal disease. *J. Clin. Invest.* 53:904–912, 1974.

98. Shizgal, H.M., Spanier, H., Kurtz, R.S. Effect of parenteral nutrition on body composition in the critically ill patient. *Am. J. Surg.* 131:156–161, 1976.

99. Shils, M.E., Burke, A.W., Greene, H.L., et al. Guidelines for essential trace element preparations for parenteral use. *J.A.M.A.* 241:2051–2054, 1979.

100. Haver, E.C., Kaminski, M.V. Trace metal profile of parenteral nutrition solutions. *Am. J. Clin. Nutr.* 31:264–268, 1978.

101. Robinson, L.A., Mabry, C.D., Wright, B.T. Vitamin regimens in parenteral nutrition: A dilemma. *J.P.E.N.* 6:76–77, 1982.

102. McClain, C.J. Trace metal abnormalities in adults during hyperalimentation. *J.P.E.N.* 5:424–429, 1981.

103. Wilmore, D.W., Moylan, J.A., Helmkamp, G.M., Pruitt, B.A. Clinical evaluation of a 10% intravenous fat emulsion for parenteral nutrition in thermally injured patients. *Ann. Surg.* 178:503–513, 1973.

104. Jeejeebhoy, K.N., Anderson, G.H., Nakhooda, A.F., et al. Metabolic studies in total parenteral nutrition with lipid in man. *J. Clin. Invest.* 57:125–136, 1976.

105. Kien, C., Browning, C., Jona, J., Starshak, R.J. Rickets in premature infants receiving parenteral nutrition: A case report and review of the literature. *J.P.E.N.* 6:152–156, 1982.

106. Kishi, H., Yamiji, A., Kataoka, K., et al. Vitamin A and E requirements during total parenteral nutrition. *J.P.E.N.* 5:420–423, 1981.

107. Stromberg, P., Shenkin, A., Campbell, R.A., et al. Vitamin status during total parenteral nutrition. *J.P.E.N.* 5:295–299, 1981.

108. Richardson, T.J., Sgoutas, D. Essential fatty acid deficiency in four adult patients during total parenteral nutrition. *Am. J. Clin. Nutr.* 28:258–263, 1975.

109. Fleming, C.R., Smith, L.M., Hodges, R.E. Essential fatty acid deficiency in adults receiving total parenteral nutrition. *Am. J. Clin. Nutr.* 29:976–983, 1976.

110. Fischer, J.E., Rosen, H.M., Ebeid, A.M., et al. The effect of normalization of plasma amino acids on hepatic encephalopathy in man. *Surgery* 80:77–91, 1976.

111. Rossi-Fanelli, F., Angelico, M., Cangiano, C., et al. Effect of glucose and/or branched chain amino acid infusion on plasma amino acid imbalance in chronic liver failure. *J.P.E.N.* 5:414–419, 1981.

112. Abel, R.M., Beck, C.H., Abbott, W.M., et al. Improved survival from acute renal failure after treatment with intravenous essential L-amino acids and glucose. *N. Engl. J. Med.* 288:695–699, 1973.

113. Wilmore, W.D., Dudrick, S.J. Treatment of acute renal failure with intravenous essential L-amino acids. *Arch. Surg.* 99:669–673, 1969.

114. Ivey, M., Riella, M., Mueller, W., Scribner, B. Long-term parenteral nutrition in the home. *Am. J. Hosp. Pharm.* 32:1032–1036, 1975.

115. Shils, M.E. A program for total parenteral nutrition at home. *Am. J. Clin. Nutr.* 28:1429–1435, 1976.

116. Jeejeebhoy, K.N., Zohrab, W.J., Langer, B., et al. Total parenteral nutrition at home for 23 months, without complication and with good rehabilitation. *Gastroenterology* 65:811–820, 1973.

117. Dudrick, S.J., Englert, DeA.M., Barroso, A.O., et al. Update on ambulatory home hyperalimentation. *Nutr. Supp. Serv.* 1:18–21, 1981.

118. Wretlind, A. Evaluation of carbohydrates in parenteral nutrition. *Nutr. Metab.* 18(Suppl. 1):242–255, 1975.

119. Young, E.A., Fletcher, J.T., Cioletti, L.A., et al. Metabolism of parenteral glucose oligosaccharides in man. *J.P.E.N.* 5:369–377, 1981.

120. Blackburn, G.L. Peripheral intravenous feeding with isotonic amino acid solutions. *Am. J. Surg.* 125:447–454, 1973.

121. Greenberg, G.R., Marliss, E.B., Anderson, G.H., et al. Protein-sparing therapy in postoperative patients. *N. Engl. J. Med.* 294:1411–1416, 1976.

122. Collins, J.P., Oxby, C.B., Hill, G.L. Intravenous amino acids and intravenous hyperalimentation as protein-sparing therapy after major surgery. A controlled clinical trial. *Lancet* 1:788–791, 1978.

123. Deitel, M., Kaminsky, V. Total nutrition by peripheral vein: The lipid system. *Can. Med. Assoc. J.* 111:152–153, 1976.

124. Hansen, L.M., Hardie, W.R., Hidalgo, J. Fat emulsion for intravenous administration: Clinical experience with Intralipid 10%. *Ann. Surg.* 184:80–88, 1976.

125. Goodgame, J.T., Jr. A critical assessment of the indications for total parenteral nutrition. *Surg. Gynecol. Obstet.* 151:433–441, 1980.

126. Burke, J.F., Wolfe, R.R., Mullany, C.J., et al. Glucose requirements following burn injury: Parameters of optional glucose infusion and possible hepatic and respiratory abnormalities following excessive glucose intake. *Ann. Surg.* 190:274–285, 1979.

127. Askanazi, J., Carpenteir, Y.A., Elwyn, D.H., et al. Influence of total parenteral nutrition on fuel utilization in injury and sepsis. *Ann. Surg.* 191:40–46, 1980.

128. Elwyn, D.H., Kinney, J.M., Jeevanandam, M., et al. Influence of increasing carbohydrate intake on glucose kinetics in injured patients. *Ann. Surg.* 190:117–127, 1979.

129. Cerra, F.B., Siegel, J.H., Coleman, B., et al. Septic autocannibalism: A failure of exogenous nutritional support. *Ann. Surg.* 192:570–579, 1980.

Discussion

Questions were presented by the audience to the panel of speakers, which consisted of Dr. DeLuca, Dr. Graham, and Dr. Young. The discussion covered a broad range of topics. The principal concern of the audience, however, was with calcium metabolism, particularly in the elderly.

It was stated clearly that adequate calcium intake and vitamin D intake during childhood do not prevent osteoporosis in later years. Nor has a clear dietary treatment been identified to deal with osteogenesis imperfecta. Some studies have reported success in dealing with osteogenesis imperfecta by stimulating collagen formation with glucocorticoids, but no clear data are available. Calcium and bone metabolism is an ongoing process and must be supported throughout life. The appearance of osteoporosis, particularly in post-menopausal women, is due to their inability to maintain bone mass. Supplemental calcium intake, 1–2 g/day, is a suggested but not proven means of management. It is also clear that estrogen, taken very early after menopause, is a proven effective treatment in prevention of bone loss and osteoporosis. However, this treatment may be accompanied by an increase in the incidence of uterine cancer if estrogens are used noncyclically and without progestational agents to allow for periodic endometrial shedding. An effective and safe means of increasing bone density is exercise. Prior to menopause, exercise results in increased calcium deposition in bone, whereas after menopause calcium loss from bone is reduced.

In the elderly patient, especially the Caucasian woman, the treatment of osteoporosis may become necessary. The most desirable situation would be identification of the subclinical stages of osteoporosis. However, current methodology precludes this approach even though the population at high risk is known. On an experimental basis, osteoporosis has been treated with 50 mg per day of oral sodium fluoride for a period of six months. About half of the patients so treated cannot tolerate sodium fluoride due to gastric disturbance, and of the remaining half, only 50 percent respond to the treatment. Those that do respond show increased trabecular volume and reduced fracture incidence.

When it becomes necessary, adequate calcium supplementation can be achieved with the least expensive calcium salt available, calcium carbonate. Other calcium salts, such as gluconate and lactate, add bulky anions which increase the total mass. Chelated calcium does not appear to be readily absorbed and is considerably more expensive than calcium carbonate. The underlying concern with dietary calcium supplementation is the possibility of inhibition of calciotropic hormones, and bone remodeling may be markedly slowed.

Further clarification was sought by the audience concerning the dosage of vitamin D supplementation. For patients who have adequate ability to convert vitamin D to the active form, 200 units per day is adequate. However, it must be borne in mind that very little is known about human vitamin D requirements at different stages of life. The recommended daily allowance of 200 or 400 units is very poorly supported by data. Inded, as little as 50 units per day may cause children to grow and to calcify normally.

On occasion, patients may indicate vitamin D resistance. Historically, patients with vitamin D–resistant rickets have been treated with 50,000 units per day. Since the nature of the defect in this disease is now known, such treatment is no longer appropriate. Nevertheless, if such patients show rickets, cautious increases in ordinary vitamin D supplementation in consultation with a bone expert may be the preferred treatment.

A somewhat different problem is presented by low-birth-weight, premature infants. These babies often have hypocalcemia and disturbed calcium metabolism. Giving them additional vitamin D is not going to help because they lack the enzymes required for vitamin D metabolism. They also lack the ability to make mature parathyroid hormone. Thus, numerous problems contribute to the hypocalcemia. Eventually, however, these patients will overcome their retarded mineralization provided they are given normal nutritional support in all other respects.

A converse problem was pointed out by calling attention to the high concentrations of calcium in certain infant formulas. Whether such formulas will have an adverse effect in premature infants will depend on their calcium absorption mechanism. Usually, however, such premature infants lack the ability to make vitamin D compounds and to hydroxylate vitamin D intermediates, and thus the problem with deficient calcium absorption is secondary.

In summarizing vitamin D requirements, the possibility of affecting parathyroid hormone and thyrocalcitonin regulatory mechanisms by the administration of vitamin D was pointed out. Furthermore, in light of the possibility of hypersensitivity to vitamin D resulting in idiopathic hypercalcemia, high daily doses of vitamin D should be avoided; no one should take more than 400 units of vitamin D per day unless prescribed by a physician for a specific disorder.

The possibility of prevention of cancer by dietary manipulation was discussed with considerable interest. Several vitamins and trace minerals were suggested by the audience as possible factors that might change cancer risk. The general consensus emerged that it would be inappropriate at this time to attempt to modify cancer risk by taking vitamin pills—a balanced diet was seen as more beneficial. Nevertheless, several substances were mentioned that are currently being studied. A trial study with carotene will be under way shortly, and retinol may be another candidate for an epidemiologic study. Retinoids, chemically related to vitamin A, are being examined by the National Cancer Institute as possible agents to reduce the incidence of certain cancers in high-risk patients. However, the danger of vitamin A toxicity must be underscored, and some epithelial tumors are actually stimulated by excess vitamin A in animals.

It appears that results are conflicting and inconclusive regarding the use of vitamin C for treatment of established tumors. For example, tumor-bearing animals receiving vitamin C dietary supplement have shown increased survival; presumably, this is due to high rates of vitamin C utilization by the tumors, and increased dietary availability of vitamin C reduces the demand on body stores. On the other hand, patients with confirmed cancers who received vitamin C in a clinical trial had no difference in survival rate from those who received a placebo.

In general, the panel stressed repeatedly the importance of an adequate, balanced diet as a primary priority. Use of vitamins or trace metals (e.g., selenium) for the reduction in risk or prevention of onset of cancer is still being evaluated.

It was pointed out that hospitals are becoming increasingly aware of the role of diet in the well-being of patients and in their recovery from disease. With increasing frequency, hospitals are funding interdisciplinary team approaches to the management of nutritional problems of hospitalized patients. This approach has been shown to pay for itself in private hospitals.

There is a need for physicians to better their understanding of nutrition. This need might be satisfied by more thorough and systematic teaching in medical schools, by greater dissemination of information from the Department of Agriculture and other agencies, by more widespread publication of nutrition books, and by conferences, workshops, and continuing medical education programs on nutrition. The necessity for such efforts is underscored by the recognition that a minimum of 30 percent of hospitalized patients are malnourished. All of these efforts, which appear to be on the increase, should strengthen the awareness of physicians of the importance of nutrition.

III Nutrition and Growth in the Young

8 Obesity in Adulthood and Predisposition of Children Toward Obesity

Roslyn B. Alfin-Slater, Ph.D.

Human society has always had its cases of obesity, which tends to become a problem in all countries as soon as the threat of starvation is removed by increases in available food supplies. Obesity knows no age, sex, or racial boundaries. Probably the best definition of obesity is that it is an excessive accumulation of adipose tissue in the body. The fat cells, or adipocytes, which constitute adipose tissue, appear to have as their exclusive function the formation, retention, and mobilization of fat within the cell membrane. The word *adipose* is actually derived from the Greek *aedeps* meaning "lard," the adipose tissue of pigs. And adiposity implies that there is an excess of fat in adipocytes as well as an increased number of cells. In the nineteenth century the term *obesity* came into common usage, with the implication that excess adiposity might be a metabolic disorder.

Composition of Adipocytes

Human adipose tissue is derived from both endogenous and exogenous sources. It is well known that when food is ingested in excess of caloric need, regardless of whether these excess calories are eaten as carbohydrate, protein, or fat, the excess calories are converted to triglycerides, primarily in the liver and in adipose tissue, which are then deposited in the adipose tissue depots. The liver also contributes to adipose tissue stores by forming triglycerides from fatty acids resulting from the digestion of dietary fat. Therefore, although foods rich in carbohydrate and fat are thought of as "fattening" foods, it is scientifically incorrect to single out these foods for this incriminating label. Any food or combination of foods, if eaten in excess of caloric demands, will be "fattening." However, because carbohydrate foods are usually less expensive and are present in foods that are particularly appealing to most people, they are the ones that are commonly eaten in excess. Normal, healthy people usually have no digestive problems with carbohydrate-containing foods, which are easily digested and metabolized to supply energy for daily activities.

Value of Adipose Tissue

Adipose tissue is a very valuable resource. It is the source of energy in times of food deprivation. The ability of people to survive in periods of starvation depends on their ability to mobilize sources of energy within the body—that is, to produce glucose from glycogen, amino acids from protein, and fatty acids from triglycerides. There are only meager deposits of glycogen (0.2 kg) in muscle and liver, sufficient to supply 800 calories, which would be exhausted in a rather short period of time; and not too much more is available as a potential energy source in the form of protein (6 kg, equivalent to 24,000 calories) in these and other tissues. Since the storage of calories as glycogen and protein necessitates the accumulation of two to four times their weight of water as a diluent, each gram of these stored nutrients in tissue provides only approximately 2 calories. On the other hand, triglycerides in adipose tissue may comprise as much as 95 percent of the tissue weight, and therefore one gram of tissue may yield approximately 9 calories.

Normal individuals store approximately 15 kg of triglyceride; obese individuals store considerably more depending on the degree of obesity. Fortunately, people depend on stored lipids during periods of calorie deprivation.

Two different types of adipose tissue have now been recognized, white fat and brown fat. An interesting development in the study of obesity concerns the function of this brown fat in the body. Brown fat is found in the neck, around the kidneys and adrenal glands, and around the aorta. When the body is exposed to a cold environment, the white fat insulates the body but the brown fat actually supplies heat, and therefore fat calories are consumed in this process.

Effects of Excess Adipose Tissue on Disease Incidence and Organ Systems

When adipose tissue is present in excess, it has adverse effects on a number of organs; it limits the productivity of individuals and populations and contributes to increased susceptibility to many diseases—diabetes, hypertension, gallbladder disease, gout, degenerative arthritis, skin ailments, and possibly cardiovascular disease [1]. For each extra pound of fat, 15–25 miles of blood vessels must be provided, resulting in an extra burden on the heart. Obese people also have many postsurgical problems and obstetrical difficulties, and they have been found to be more susceptible to accidents and to certain types of cancer, for example, uterine cancer.

Measurement of Obesity

Obesity is the leading form of malnutrition in affluent nations. It is estimated that in the United States between 40 and 80 million people are considered obese. Obesity can be determined by several methods, some more precise than others [1]. These include measurement of whole body potassium content to measure lean body mass or measurements of bone, muscle, and fat widths by roentgenography of the extremities. The skinfold thickness is an indication of the amount of subcutaneous fat measured in several places, such as the upper arm, using a special type of calipers. Usually measurements of more than one inch indicate some degree of obesity. Measurement of the body circumference at various sites has also been used to determine body fat. The life insurance weight for height tables, which give average values, are probably the most widely used reference. Less precise but useful methods include measurement of waist and chest: if the circumference of the waist is greater than that of the chest, this is an indication of excess abdominal fat. A ruler test is performed lying flat with a ruler placed on the abdomen. If the ruler does not touch both the ribs and the pelvis, the person is carrying too much weight. The final test is the mirror test.

The Question of Desirable Weight

The problem that remains is to determine what is desirable weight. It has been suggested that the desirable weight for women can be calculated as follows: for a height of 60 inches (5 feet) the desirable weight is 100 pounds; for each additional inch 5 pounds should be added. For men, the 60-inch weight should be 106 pound, with 6 pounds to be added for each additional inch in height. If the body weight is 20 percent in excess of the desirable weight, the individual is probably obese.

Obesity in Children

Obesity in children is often the precursor of obesity in adults [2]. Whether childhood obesity is inherited or whether it results from overeating and physical inactivity is still being debated [1–3]. It is known that children who are prone to obesity are usually larger than the average for their age, with larger bones and heavier muscles [2,4]. Fat babies usually have larger and more numerous fat cells than do normal-weight babies [3,5].

Obesity that occurs in families may be partly inherited, but in many cases it is probably a result of simple conditioning of eating habits during infancy and childhood [3]. Although the breast-fed baby can regulate his or her intake of milk, the amount of nourishment consumed by the bottle-fed baby is controlled by whoever feeds him or her. Parents who fear that their babies will be undernourished will use all sorts of methods of persuasion to ensure that the last ounce of fluid in the bottle is ingested [3,6]. The seeds of obesity are sown early in childhood, since the eating habits of children are influenced by those of their parents. Approximately 80 percent of obese children become obese adults [2].

Adipocytes: Cell Size versus Cell Number

Obesity or adiposity can occur through an increase in adipose cell number, cell size, or both [3]. It has been reported that the number of adipocytes can be increased at certain critical times during the life cycle—the first occurring from birth to 2 years of age and the second at puberty [4,5]. There is some evidence that very obese children also continue to increase the number of fat cells between the age of 2 and puberty. Recent evidence suggests that the number of adipose cells can be increased in adults if the weight gain is sufficiently high, since the number of cells increases when the size of adipocytes reaches a maximum limit [1,5]. However, when weight is lost there is a decrease in cell size but not in number, which is one of the reasons that lost weight is regained so easily.

Explanations for Obesity

Many possible explanations for obesity have been examined [1], including abnormalities in the assimilation and metabolism of food, possibly related to hormonal changes that may include a reduced ability of the body to respond to insulin; a decreased production of thyroid hormone; and interference with the proper functioning of hypothalamic regulation of appetite. It has been found that even grossly obese persons have normal basal metabolic rates. Nor is there an alteration of the efficiency in the use of food by the obese during exercise or digestion. However, there does seem to be some disorder of appetite regulatory mechanisms involved in obesity. The hypothalamus controls not only the sensation of hunger but also the feeling of satiety. This latter sensation is not an immediate reaction to the presence of sufficient food in the stomach but one that is delayed, which therefore can result in the ingestion of more food than the body requires. If the hypothalamus is injured, appetite control is affected, and excess eating will be accompanied by excess deposits in adipose tissues as a result [1]. In some cases, even when the hypothalamus is intact and is in control of appetite, the individual may not pay attention to the message that the brain sends, and he or she overeats in spite of the body's attempt to regulate food intake.

There is also a cultural determinant of proper weight; important factors are a person's appearance, environmental factors, and the sight, smell, and taste of food. Stresses such as anxiety, fatigue, boredom, jealousy, and tension can also result in overeating.

Reducing Diets

The nation as a whole seems to be preoccupied with a host of diets to relieve overweight. There are reducing diets low in carbohydrates, high in carbohydrates, low in protein, high in protein, or high in fiber. There are diet regimens that recommend limited foods or strange combinations of foods. None of these is without potential risk [1,7]. The low-carbohydrate diet can result in ketosis and disturbance in the acid-base balance of the body, as well as in high uric acid levels that may cause gout in susceptible individuals. The "protein-sparing" diets have resulted in potassium depletion and cardiac arrhythmias. Fruit and high-fiber diets have caused diarrhea and trace mineral malabsorption. Fortunately, in most cases these "quick-weight-loss" diets are so monotonous and restrictive that adherence is difficult. The consistent failure rate associated with such diets is estimated to be over 80 percent. For those who do achieve a weight loss, in many cases it is not sustained.

Obesity is not simply remedied. The "cure," which involves ingesting fewer calories than are expended, also involves a change in life-style with the introduction of a continuing exercise program [1,4]. The prevention of obesity is much more successful than the remedy.

Summary

Excess caloric intake, regardless of its source from protein, carbohydrate, or fat, is converted to triglycerides and stored in adipose tissue. This represents a valuable potential source of energy substrate in time of need. However, in obesity, when adipose tissue is present in excess, adverse effects are experienced on a number of organs, and increased susceptibility to certain diseases results. Several means of measurement of obesity have been discussed.

Obesity in children is often the precursor of obesity in adults. Both genetic factors and learned eating habits in childhood may be responsible for adult obesity. The number of adipocytes has been reported to increase at certain critical times in life. When weight is lost, there is a decrease in cell size but not in number.

Several hypotheses have been advanced to explain obesity. Among these should be mentioned alterations of the hormonal milieu and responsiveness and changes in appetite control. This question remains, however, to be resolved.

In general, specific reducing diets are not regarded as a satisfactory means of control of obesity. The most desirable method of body weight control is reduced caloric intake combined with a continuing exercise program.

References

1. Stern, J.S., Kane-Nussen, B., Obesity: Its assessment, risks and treatments. In Hodges, R.E. (Ed.), *Human Nutrition: A Comprehensive Treatise*, vol. 4, *Nutrition: Metabolic and Clinical Applications*. New York: Plenum Press, 1979. Pp. 347–407.
2. Charney, E., Goodman, H., McBridge, M., et al. Childhood antecedents of adult obesity. *N. Engl. J. Med.* 296:6–9, 1976.
3. Winick, M. Childhood obesity. *Nutrition Today* 9:6–12, 1974.
4. Knittle, J.L. Obesity in childhood: A problem in adipose tissue development. *J. Pediatr.* 81:1048–1049, 1972.
5. Brook, C. Evidence for a sensitive period in adipose-cell replication in man. *Lancet* 2:624–627, 1972.
6. Himes, J.H. Infant feeding practices and obesity. *J. Am. Diet. Assoc.* 75:122–127, 1979.
7. Hegsted, D.M. Rating the diets. *Health* 15:21–32, 1983.

Suggested Reading

Berland, T., and the editors of *Consumer's Guide*. *Rating the diets '83*. New York: Signet, 1983.

9 Protein-Energy Malnutrition

Patrick V.J. Hegarty, Ph.D.

The terms *protein-energy malnutrition* (PEM) and *protein-calorie malnutrition* (PCM) have become synonymous with reduced growth and development of infants and young children, especially in developing countries. Recent evidence has indicated an involvement of a larger segment of the population. The prevalence of severe PEM probably exceeds 15 percent in many acute-care hospitals in the United States [1]. It is not confined to diseases such as cancer but is widely distributed over broad disease categories. Detection of patients at nutritional risk is important because of (1) the association between impaired nutrition and an increased risk of complications, and (2) the availability of enteral and parenteral feeding techniques. The proportion of malnourished patients who are elderly has not been documented but is considered to be relatively high [2]. This presents some difficulty in the characterization of PEM. The physical, anatomic, and biochemical changes that occur during aging indicate that measurements traditionally made to detect the presence of PEM may be inappropriate for the elderly due to a lack of specific norms for comparison [2]. Therefore, it is acknowledged that PEM may be a problem in some elderly people and in some hospitalized patients in the United States. The remainder of this chapter is devoted to the problems caused by PEM in the young child.

Definition

Three clinical types of severe PEM have been recognized: kwashiorkor, marasmus, and marasmic kwashiorkor. Since the distinction between these types is based on clinical findings, the classification tends to be qualitative and subjective. A refinement was introduced in 1970 by the Wellcome classification [3], which is based on the presence or absence of edema and a deficit in body weight (Table 9-1). Children with edema and weighing between 60 and 80 percent of their expected weight for age were classified as having kwashiorkor; children without edema and weighing less than 60 percent of their expected weight for age were classified as having marasmus; and children with edema and a body weight less than 60 percent of the expected weight for age were considered to have marasmic kwashiorkor. Children without edema and weighing between 60 and 80 percent of their expected weight for age were

Table 9–1
The Wellcome Classification of Protein-Energy Malnutrition

Body Weight (% of Standard)[a]	*Edema*	
	Present	*Absent*
80–60	Kwashiorkor	Underweight
<60	Marasmic kwashiorkor	Marasmus

Source: Data taken from Alleyne et al. [3].
[a]Standard = fiftieth centile Boston value.

classified as underweight. However, this classification cannot be applied when the age of the child is unknown, and it does not take into account the chronicity of the disease process. Furthermore, the designation of the extent of the edema is frequently subjective. There are considerable technical difficulties in the accurate measurement of total body water and extracellular fluid volume [4].

Prevalence

Malnutrition has been recognized for centuries in infants in Europe and later in North America, usually taking the form of marasmus. In a controversial article, McLaren [5] traced the history of severe undernutrition in children, starting with the pioneering work of Cicely Williams in the Gold Coast (now called Ghana) in 1932. McLaren's paper and the subsequent correspondence in the *Lancet* illustrate the problems involved in placing the prevalence of PEM in historical perspective. A recent paper [6] indicates that approximately 434 million people (25 percent prevalence) in developing countries can be classified as "undernourished." Comparable values for developed regions are 28 million people (3 percent prevalence). It must be reemphasized that undernutrition is not confined to the developing regions of the world. A further important point is that daily energy supply per person, expressed as a percentage of requirement, is 107 percent for the entire world. Therefore, the problem is not the supply of food energy but its global distribution.

Protein-energy malnutrition occurs in varying degrees of severity. Behar, in a paper entitled "What is marginal malnutrition?" [7], refers to surveys on the prevalence of PEM in developing countries which showed that only 1 to 3 percent of the children suffered from severe PEM, whereas at least ten times that percentage had less severe forms. The prevalence may be greater in males: boys were more severely affected by starvation in German orphanages after World War II [8].

General Clinical Features

The following classification has been taken from Alleyne and colleagues [3].

1. *Kwashiorkor.* This syndrome is found predominantly in older infants and young children whose requirements for protein and energy have not been met for some time. The children are apathetic, irritable, weak, and inactive, and have edema and a fatty liver. Changes in hair and skin, hepatomegaly, and hypothermia are seen frequently. Serum albumin is reduced, and anemia is nearly always present. Vitamin A deficiency is seen in some parts of the world. Anorexia, intermittent diarrhea, and vomiting after eating are common complaints.

2. *Marasmus.* Gross wasting of muscle and subcutaneous tissue, marked stunting, and no detectable edema are the main characteristics of marasmus. The highest incidence is in infancy. The infant is usually irritable, and appetite is often good. Hypothermia, motor retardation, and weakness are common. Hair and skin changes are less pronounced and less common than in kwashiorkor. Regional and geographic variations occur in the three forms of PEM, and the reader is referred to other sources for details [3,5].

3. *"Wasting" versus "stunting".* The criterion used by the World Health Organization in defining PEM is a deficit in weight for age. Waterlow [9] has argued that this is a bad indicator because it confuses two physiologically distinct effects, deficit in weight for height (wasting) and deficit in height for age (stunting). He then concludes that stunting is the commonest form of undernutrition; that smallness in physical size is, in itself, of little importance; that smallness is accompanied by mental and behavioral handicaps; and that these handicaps are in large degree the result not of malnutrition but of social deprivation. He has indicated that if stunting is unimportant, and if the definition of malnutrition were based only on deficit of weight for height, then the estimated number of malnourished children in the world would be

Table 9–2
Proportion of Malnourished Children in Nepal and Sri Lanka

	Children in Sample Described as Malnourished (%)	
Criterion of Malnutrition	*Nepal*	*Sri Lanka*
Wasted,[a] stunted,[b] wasted and stunted	56.2	38.1
Wasted, wasted and stunted	7.3	6.7

Source: Data taken from Waterlow [10].
[a]Defined as less than 80 percent of reference median.
[b]Defined as less than 90 percent of reference median.

reduced by 80 percent (Table 9-2). He cautions, however, that these children would still be underprivileged, and that their condition therefore should not be considered satisfactory. The natural history of stunting—its causes and sequelae—is a subject that should be given top priority in nutritional science [10]. If his argument is correct, then, Waterlow concludes that measures to combat malnutrition, such as feeding programs, will not have much effect unless at the same time they reduce the extent of social deprivation. Furthermore, the extent of undernutrition will vary considerably depending on which parameter is used to define undernutrition.

Dietary Factors

In the 1950s kwashiorkor was thought to be caused by a deficient intake of protein while energy intake was adequate. Marasmus was thought to result from a lack of both protein and energy. By the end of the 1960s the distinction in the etiology of kwashiorkor and marasmus was not this simple. The reasons for this change in diagnosis are given elsewhere [3]. One undisputed dietary factor in the development of both types of PEM is the duration of breast feeding; the elimination of breast feeding leads on to the problems caused by environmental factors.

Environmental Factors

Mata [11] reviews literature indicating that malnutrition does not occur among wild animals living in small population groups. Ancestral man organized in small groups of hunters and gatherers did not suffer from endemic malnutrition as it is observed today in developing nations. The location (latitude) and climate of a given territory have been important determinants of malnutrition. Mata also reviews macroenvironment and microenvironment (home) factors in the development of malnutrition and infection [11].

Diarrhea may be the commonest disease/symptom in the world [12]. In Central America a majority of childhood deaths are associated with diarrhea. Morbidity from diarrheal disease must be measured not only in terms of the life-threatening effects of water and electrolyte loss, dehydration, and sepsis, but also in terms of the impact on growth and nutrition in children under the age of 5. Diarrhea may cause malabsorption of various nutrients, including sugars, fats, nitrogen, and amino acids. Extensive studies on the effect of diarrhea on vitamin and trace element absorption are not available. However, malabsorption of vitamin B_{12}, folate, vitamin A, and zinc have been reported [12]. Recent evidence indicates that we cannot quantify the nutritional cost of infections. Furthermore, we remain for the most part unable to predict the

Table 9–3
Interventions That Will Improve Nutrition and Health

Intervention	*Effect*
Water supply and control of excreta	Prevention of food loss and nutrient wastage due to diarrhea and parasitism
Immunoprophylaxis	Prevention of anorexia and nutrient wastage due to measles, whooping cough, and other childhood diseases
Maternal technology	Prevention of infection in children; improvement of child nutrition; increase in child survival
Family planning	Delayed conception; increase in childspacing; improvement of maternal and fetal nutrition
Agricultural measures	Increased food production; prevention of food loss

Source: Adapted from Mata [11].

relative nutritional benefit of a given package of health or "nutrition" intervention [13]. It would seem prudent, however, to follow the interventions that will improve nutrition and health (Table 9-3) as outlined by Mata [11].

Although diarrhea presents major nutritional problems to the child, one study showed that deworming of intestinal helminth parasites did not change the absorption of nitrogen, carbohydrates, and fats in children [14]. Nitrogen balance and net protein utilization (NPU) were not affected by the parasites. This is an interesting recent observation that requires further investigation.

Metabolic Studies: The Pathogenesis of Adaptation to Kwashiorkor and Marasmus

It has been realized that the changes that occur in PEM are not simply impaired or disturbed functions. In 1968 John Waterlow proposed the concept of adaptation in the child to an environment ranging from hostile to suboptimal. This has been considered to be a major contribution to the understanding of nutrition and malnutrition.

Various adaptations in PEM have been reviewed [3]. Following restriction of either protein or total energy, there were reductions in the mass of the intestine, villous height, protein and DNA content, mitosis and cell migration rates, and disaccharidase and dipeptidase content. Adaptations to low blood sugar, anemia, and energy utilization also occur in PEM [3]. A reduction in capacity for digestion and absorption is a normal response of animals and man to a reduced intake. Evidence for adaptation in neurons in PEM has been obtained. The silent and apathetic immobility of the acutely malnourished child is an extreme example of adaptive mechanisms. Malnutrition retards growth and maturation, and it may be that animals who cannot adapt by reducing these two activities do not survive.

An extensive review of the literature on whether there are health hazards to children who are underweight and underheight for age concludes that we should be cautious in accepting the widely held view that children are malnourished or at greater risk because they fail to reach maximum growth potential, or to conform to growth standards [15].

Energy Metabolism

In 1968 Gopalan introduced the term *dysadaptation* to the study of kwashiorkor. He indicated that the biochemical mechanisms usually involved in the protection of tissues like liver at the expense of less essential muscle during energy deficit failed to operate in some children, and thus they developed kwashiorkor. Impairment in hormonal control via insulin, cortisol, and growth hormone is considered to be important in the differential genesis of kwashiorkor and marasmus [3]. However, these considerations may be academic because clear-cut cases of marasmus or kwashiorkor are rare.

Edema

A decrease in serum albumin in PEM has long been considered to be the factor in causing edema. However, nutritional edema can occur in the absence of hypoalbuminemia. Patrick [16] concludes that other mechanisms, possibly involving trace elements and the ratio of cholesterol to phospholipid, may be responsible for alteration in cell permeability.

Endocrine Changes

Most studies have reported low fasting levels of plasma insulin in PEM. The reason for this is unclear. Among the possible reasons are low food intake, pancreatic atrophy, beta-cell damage leading to poor insulin secretion and impaired glucose tolerance in severe PEM, and chromium deficiency [17]. Plasma cortisol concentrations are elevated in PEM, particularly when there is a high degree of wasting. Infection and hypoglycemia are considered the prime factors for this increase. Reports concerning the plasma levels of growth hormone in severe PEM are frequently conflicting; the concentrations may be different in kwashiorkor and marasmus. Whitehead and Lunn [17] conclude that when a child has insufficient intake of food, exactly which organ is affected the most is a reflection of the overall hormonal status of the child.

Mineral Deficiencies

Much research remains to be done on the extent of mineral deficiencies in PEM. Because of the poor quality of the diet and the malabsorption caused by diarrhea, it is probable that most minerals are affected by PEM. There is a net deficit of potassium, and depletion of magnesium, iron, and zinc have been reported extensively. Total body sodium is increased, and there are alterations in the sodium pump [3,16].

Is There a Protein Crisis?

McLaren [5] considers that the concept of the much publicized world protein "gap," "crisis," or "problem" arose from the description of kwashiorkor in Africa in the 1930s, and from the assumption, which was wrong, that malnutrition in children occurs as kwashiorkor throughout the world. Emphasis is now also given to the energy content of the diet. The general consensus today is that there is a shortage of food in certain parts of the world.

Treatment of PEM

Some children with PEM die within a few days after hospital admission because of inadequate or misguided treatment [18]. Furthermore, recovery from PEM is unnecessarily slow in some hospitals. Treatment of children with PEM can be divided into the acute phase, involving resuscitation and initiation of cure, and the rehabilitation phase, involving catch-up growth and transfer to a family-type diet. Children are most at risk in the acute phase, and therefore treatment during this period is best carried out in the hospital [18].

The most life-threatening conditions during the acute phase/resuscitation are infections, anemia, severe dehydration, and errors in assessing the adequacy of rehydration (errors should be on the side of underhydration). Other problems requiring treatment are magnesium and vitamin A deficiencies, hypoglycemia, and hypothermia. During the acute phase/initiation of cure, oral feeding is introduced and diarrhea is eliminated. This stage is usually completed within a week of admission [18].

The rehabilitation phase/catch-up growth requires attention not only to the quantity and quality of protein in the diet but also to high-energy intakes, which are necessary for rapid catch-up growth. A high-energy milk formula in which the energy density of milk is doubled by adding vegetable oil is successful [18]. The rehabilitation phase/transfer to family-type diet occurs when the child is ready for discharge. The diet is based on the multimix principle, which is a nutritious mixture of low-cost foods.

Use of Experimental Animals in Replicating PEM

Unfortunately, there are problems in the interpretation of data pertaining to PEM when experimental animals are used. There are differences in physiology and biochemistry, in the time scale of the undernutrition, in the timing of the birth event in relation to maturity, and in the contour of the growth curve [3]. Nevertheless, animals have provided valuable information [19,20].

Summary

Protein-energy malnutrition has always been associated with infants and children, especially in developing countries. Recent evidence indicates that PEM may be a problem among some hospitalized or elderly people in the United States. PEM is a complex nutritional problem that requires particular attention to the quality and quantity of diet during rehabilitation. A deficit in protein and/or energy is compounded by a low intake and/or malabsorption of minerals and vitamins. A major contributing factor to malabsorption of nutrients in infants is infections, especially diarrhea. Therefore, the correction of health problems caused by PEM in these circumstances requires attention to the social environment as well as to the quality of the diet.

References

1. Blackburn, G.L., Harvey, K.B. Prognostic strength of nutritional assessment. In Harper, A.E., Davis, G.K. (Eds.), *Nutrition in Health and Disease and International Development. Symposia from the Twelfth International Congress of Nutrition.* New York: Alan R. Liss, 1981. Pp. 689–697.

2. Mitchell, C.O., Lipschitz, D.A. Detection of protein-calorie malnutrition in the elderly. *Am. J. Clin. Nutr.* 35:398–406, 1982.

3. Alleyne, G.A.O., Hay, R.W., Picou, D.I., et al. *Protein-Energy Malnutrition.* London: E. Arnold, 1977.

4. Patrick, J., Reeds, P.J., Jackson, A.A., et al. Total body water in malnutrition: The possible role of energy intake. *Br. J. Nutr.* 39:417–424, 1978.

5. McLaren, D.S. The great protein fiasco. *Lancet* 2:93–96, 1974.

6. Miller, D.S. Prevalence of nutritional problems in the world. *Proc. Nutr. Soc.* 38:197–205, 1979.

7. Behar, M. What is marginal malnutrition? In Harper, A.E., Davis, G.K., (Eds.), *Nutrition in Health and Disease and International Development. Symposia from the Twelfth International Congress of Nutrition.* New York: Alan R. Liss, 1981. Pp. 237–246.

8. Widdowson, E.M. The response of the sexes to nutritional stress. *Proc. Nutr. Soc.* 35:175–180, 1976.

9. Waterlow, J.C. Childhood malnutrition—the global problem. *Proc. Nutr. Soc.* 38:1–9, 1979.

10. Waterlow, J.C. Crisis for nutrition. *Proc. Nutr. Soc.* 40:195–207, 1981.

11. Mata, L. The malnutrition-infection complex and its environment factors. *Proc. Nutr. Soc.* 38:29–40, 1979.

12. Rosenberg, I.H., Solomons, N.W., Schneider, R.E. Malabsorption associated with diarrhea and intestinal infections. *Am. J. Clin. Nutr.* 30:1248–1253, 1977.

13. Brown, K.H., Black, R.E. The nutritional cost of infections. In Harper, A.E., Davis, G.K., (Eds.), *Nutrition in Health and Disease and International Development. Symposia from the Twelfth International Congress of Nutrition.* New York: Alan R. Liss, 1981. Pp. 467–477.

14. Ju, J.S., Hwang, W.I., Ryu, T.G. Protein absorption of pre-school children with intestinal helminth parasites. In Torun, B., Young, V.R., Rand, W.M. (Eds.), *Protein-Energy Requirements of Developing Countries: Evaluation of New Data.* Tokyo: The United Nations University, 1981. Pp. 191–201.

15. Walker, A.R.P., Walker, B.F. What is the health hazard to children who are underweight and underheight for age? *S. Afr. J. Sci.* 72:203–208, 1976.

16. Patrick, J. Oedema in protein energy malnutrition: The role of the sodium pump. *Proc. Nutr. Soc.* 38:61–68, 1979.

17. Whitehead, R.G., Lunn, P.G. Endocrines in protein-energy malnutrition. *Proc. Nutr. Soc.* 38:69–76, 1979.

18. Ashworth, A. Progress in the treatment of protein-energy malnutrition. *Proc. Nutr. Soc.* 38:89–97, 1979.

19. Kirsch, R.E., Saunders, S.J., Brock, J.F. Animal models and human protein-calorie malnutrition. *Am. J. Clin. Nutr.* 21:1225–1228, 1968.

20. Whitehead, R.G. Animal models for the study of protein-energy malnutrition. *Proc. Nutr. Soc.* 39:227–231, 1980.

10 Rebellion Against Parental Authority: Fad Diets, "Badditives," and Food Supplements

Victor Herbert, M.D., J.D.

The role of rebellion against parental authority in many of the food fads to which our young are susceptible is discussed particularly in the literature in psychiatry and sociology. Harold Morowitz of Yale has suggested that young people are vulnerable to irrational food cults because we do not teach students how to evaluate the validity of statements [1]. We do not teach epistemology and logic. We need to teach our young to ask, "How do we know the things that we know?" They should know the methodology for evaluating the validity of statements. They should be able to recognize facts from fiction, to separate the specious from the sound. What we often face in our young is self-righteous certainty about the validity of nutrition frauds because they tend to display the arrogance of ignorance [2].

A National Assessment of Education Progress, federally funded, is conducted in the United States. The last report of this study, which monitored school performance of 106,000 young people of ages 9, 13, and 17 [3], showed that the reasoning ability of our young has been progressively declining for the last ten years, with the vast majority of young people less able to separate fact from fiction, having inadequate thinking skills or ability to interpret what they read beyond a superficial level; less able to draw reasonable conclusions; and less able to assess whether something is a worthless anecdote or testimonial or rather a legitimate piece of evidence on any given subject. Testimonials and anecdotes are worthless as evidence because they do not separate cause and effect from coincidence or fact from fiction. Our young have not adequately learned how to look for evidence or to separate the wheat from the chaff in what they read. In 1983, the National Commission on Excellence in Education delivered a scathing report on the "tide of mediocrity" devastating American education. It was the cover story in *Newsweek* (May 9, 1983).

Michael Sovern, president of Columbia University, stated in his inaugural address: "We pronounce a national scandal the inability of our young to recognize, much less write, a clear sentence, but we tolerate with remarkable equanimity similar inability to know what it means to think scientifically. We pay for our ignorance with erratic swings between public policies founded first on wonder and awe and then on fear and mistrust" [4].

This research was supported by the Research Service of the U.S. Veterans Administration and USPHS Grant no. AM20526.

Nobel laureate Arthur Kornberg noted that science has fallen victim to the cultists, the misfits, and the fools because scientists have failed to explain and defend their profession. He said, "We have shrugged off rather than rejected forcefully the cultists, the misfits and the fools who erode science. Society, by ignorance, is as captive to creationists, astrologers, evangelists, food faddists and all kinds of gurus as were our ancestors held captive by fears of thunder and lightning" [5].

Nutrition quackery and nutrition faddism feed on specious slogans and beliefs that appeal to the need for control of one's own destiny and control of the environment. Quackery and faddism are based on sophistic concepts, such as the idea that natural, by definition, is good, and synthetic, by definition, is bad. This need for control is accompanied by a lack of respect for and a repudiation of knowledge, plus the perception of established experts as hated paternal authority figures, whereas promoters of quackery are seen as courageous, independent people with the foresight to penetrate the fakery of the establishment [2].

This false and destructive view of authority and of parental figures is fostered by television. Many of the entertainment shows that our young avidly watch each evening are family situations aimed at getting laughs by deriding the parental figures, making them out to be incompetent buffoons. Those most vulnerable to nutrition quackery are unable to perceive the difference betwen a genuine authority and expert—that is, someone who has earned by disciplined, controlled study, by scientific training and experience, the right to make a judgment—and people who do not follow the basic tenets of scientific canons for evaluating medical information, are not authorities, and have not earned the right to be classified as experts [6]. Many lay persons are blind to the difference between creative originality and intemperate rebelliousness and are unable to recognize the many characteristics which, when taken together, define nutrition quackery.

Our young watch television rather than read. They do not read books like Hervey Cleckley's *The Mask of Sanity*,* in which he gives a classic psychiatric explanation of cult gurus, noting that they are apparently sane, often dynamic, almost always seductive, impress others with their sincere motives and positive intentions and wind up causing great institutional and personal harm. With an unexplainable capacity to engender trust, even in experienced clinical observers, these people create chaos. The single most powerful diagnostic test, he found, was his own willingness to cash their checks. Charm, a quick sensitivity to the unspoken needs of others, and flexibility with the facts are woven into a personal charisma that entrances.

Specious logic is typical of the hypothetical questions that health gurus pose; for example, "How can you say my remedy doesn't work if you haven't tried it?" In other words, the basic scientific axiom that no remedy works

---

*Cleckley, H. *The Mask of Sanity*. St. Louis: C.V. Mosby, 1964.

until it has been demonstrated to be better than a placebo does not matter. If I tell you that cyanide cures cancer, why, you must try it! You must ignore the scientific literature which says that cyanide always kills the host at the same time it kills the tumor [2]. Our young need to learn the basic rules of epistemology as applied to fads. They need to ask, "What are the facts with relation to any claim made?" The adverse facts about starch blockers are clear-cut [7,8], but the irresponsible media do not mention them.

The irresponsible media always refer to the latest fads and frauds as a "controversy." There is no controversy. Nutrition is a science; it is not a religion. Facts are objectively ascertainable. The controversy is always a media-created one, a collision between nutrition reality and nutrition fraud in which the media say, "Let's give both sides a chance, both scientific nutrition and snake oil nutrition. Let's hear both sides. Let's give equal time to fiction. Let's be objective." It is as if, for example, we were putting on a television panel discussion on rape and felt that, in fairness to both sides, we must invite a rapist to explain why rape is really a lot of fun and should not be against the law. Or as if we were having a seminar on criminology and selected panelists from the Mafia to advise us on ethics.

It is not a question of controversy in the case of various health frauds. The scientific facts are clear, as in the case of starch blockers. Those on the market are either pure frauds and do not work at all, or if they do work, they are dangerous. It is as simple as that. The facts are that starch blockers are chemicals in beans (glycoproteins) which bind to amylase (provided they get to the amylase first, before the starch does) and which, if they work, will cause the starch to be more slowly digested and therefore to go down into the colon where it will ferment. This results in gas, which can produce nausea, abdominal pain, diarrhea, and flatus. You "get rid of your potential fat" through increased flatus, or to put it grossly, you "fart away your fat." The way to find out whether the product you are taking is a pure fraud and doesn't work at all or whether it does work and therefore is dangerous is simply to note if you are passing gas and have become socially unacceptable. If so, then the product is working and is dangerous; if not, the product is a pure fraud. It's as simple as that. But the media do not inform the public of this; they are too busy taking starch blocker advertising money.

Cults and Fads

To talk sensibly about cultism and food faddism among our young, we should define the term *cult*. Young people should learn that words have dictionary meanings. I use the term in the dictionary meaning of the word: a cult is any system for treating human sickness or preventing sickness originated by one usually claiming to have sole insight into the nature of disease, and that employs methods generally regarded as being unorthodox and unscientific

[9]. Cultists can be recognized among our young by their statement, "I believe in . . ." rather than "The evidence is that . . ." They ask speakers at meetings, "Do you believe in . . .?" rather than "What is the scientific evidence on this subject?" To "believe" in something regarding nutrition science is to engage in cult talk, not in science. Nutrition is not a religion. Religions are belief systems; science is not. To be "into" nutrition is to be involved in a belief system, not a science.

Cults relating to science have existed throughout history. For centuries there was the cult of the unicorn horn, which claimed mysterious health powers of the powdered horn. Some surveys indicate that more than a million of our young people are involved in various pseudo-religious cults, many of them food cults, which require as fundamental that one give up one's ability to think and that one accept the pronouncement of the guru as the only way to decide how to act and how to behave.

In her book *The Origins of Totalitarianism*, Hannah Arendt notes that the feelings of rootlessness, loneliness, and despair in many of the young in modern society cause those who feel adrift to seek connectedness through disciplined sets of rules, consistent even to the point of absurdity. Psychoanalyst Erich Fromm, in his book *Escape from Freedom* (a widely available paperback which many young people cannot bother to read), describes the desire to replace the complexity of real life and the uncertainties of democratic choices by a nearly childish existence in totalitarianism, in which the cult and its leaders supply all rules and all answers and a disciple meets his psychobiologic needs for relatedness by absorbing himself into the cult without true connectedness. The cultist abandons his own personality and adopts that of the cult, becoming an automaton reciting what he has been taught, for which Fromm created the phrase "automaton conformity." This lack of reality orientation at the heart of health and nutrition cults, as well as other pseudo-religious cults, makes their members dangerous to themselves and to others [2].

Nutrition is a science, not a religion. The facts about nutrition and diet can be found in many responsible publications, such as the Recommended Dietary Allowances (RDA) of the National Research Council, publications of the Department of Agriculture, and *Consumer Reports*. But our young people want snake oil nutrition, not nutrition reality.

To determine for themselves whether they are being sucked into nutrition cults, young people have only to ask themselves, "What am I being told is the way my nutrition state should be diagnosed? Are the diagnostic tests rational?" If the test is hair analysis or a Donsbach or Kelley computer questionnaire (available in thousands of health food stores and chiropractic offices around the country), then what is being promoted is questionable nutrition practice based on snake oil nutrition testing [10,11]. One can pick up any issue of the leading purveyor of nutrition misinformation to the public, *Prevention* magazine, and find full-page advertisements for hair analysis to diagnose your nutrition status. In the universities in New York City, many students are sending away $25 to $50 and getting a "delineation of their nutrition status" based on hair analysis and then taking the advice which always accompanies the report suggesting they buy a wide variety of totally unnecessary supplements, a number of which can be dangerous.

Hair analysis is worthless [10,11]. First, it is not true that it can tell a person about his vitamin status. There are no vitamins in hair above the root, so providing a vitamin status from a hair analysis is a fraud. Providing people with their mineral status by hair analysis is also largely a fraud. There is no generally accepted lower limit of normal for any mineral in hair. Any nutrition scientist who regularly reads responsible journals like the *American Journal of Clinical Nutrition* is fully aware that children with normal iron status can have so-called low hair iron and children with protein-calorie undernutrition can have normal hair copper but serious copper deficiency in their tissues [11]. Conversely, mineral-deficient children often have "normal" hair zinc, iron, or copper.

Hair is a dead tissue, not a live one. Its only value is as a late test in assessing nutrient toxicity, and therefore it is even fraudulent in that area to represent it as a better test than testing living tissues such as blood. We get rid of excesses of toxic metals by excretion through our integument (our skin, fingernails, hair). If you want to know if someone was poisoned to death as a result of having been given a little arsenic in each meal, you can get evidence on that subject by exhuming the body and demonstrating that as you go up the hair shaft there is a lot of arsenic all the way, indicating that it was steadily supplied in the diet during the months that hair was growing. However, if you want to know if someone is being poisoned with arsenic now, look in the blood where the evidence will be; hair only grows two-fifths of an inch per month, so the evidence will not be in hair an inch from the scalp until three months from now, and what is in the hair can get there from shampoos, air pollution, and a lot of other things that do not necessarily put the poison in your body [10,11]. If you are attempting to diagnose whether an inner-city child has lead poisoning (which is a real problem, because 5 percent of inner-city children in some studies have substantial lead poisoning and up to 20 percent may have lesser degrees), hair analysis is the *last* test you perform because it is the last thing that becomes abnormally high. The most sensitive test is blood lead or free erythrocyte protoporphyrin, which is regularly used to pick up early lead poisoning before the child becomes brain-damaged or neurologically disabled from lead poisoning as a result of playing in leaded automobile exhausts and eating lead-based paints and other sources of lead (including health food store dolomite and bone meal [12]).

The snake oil nutrition questionnaires that young people fill out (which are available on several college compuses in the Northeast, as I found to my chagrin) are largely fraudulent [10]. They ask a large number of questions, of which only a few are legitimately related to nutrition (questions on dietary intake); the rest are questions of the quality of "Are you tired after a hard day's work?" If you answer "Yes," the computer responds by saying that you need half the products the store or chiropractor is selling. Young people believe this because they believe that computers never lie, forgetting the basic computer maxim encompassed in the acronym GIGO—"garbage in, garbage out." If you program the computer with garbage, all you are going to get back from it is garbage. If you program the computer with the lie that you need 50 mg of extra vitamin C for every cigarette smoked, the computer will lie that the one-pack-a-day smoker needs an extra gram of vitamin C, an amount that not only can be harmful but can increase the desire to smoke, because excess vitamin C may increase nicotine craving by increasing nicotine excretion in urine. So you may get cancer faster with extra vitamin C!

Our young have to be better taught how to think. They have to be taught epistemology, the science of "how do we know the things that we know?" They have to learn to ask the fundamental questions that nutrition scientists ask of any nutrition claim: Is it effective as compared with doing nothing? Is it safe as compared with doing nothing?

Because starch blockers have not adequately answered those two questions, they were finally ordered off the market—after millions of people ingested a million tablets a day for more than a year [13]. This is the usual health food rip-off, where the public is bilked of millions of dollars for each new fad before it fades. This type of fraud is an example of the "food supplement umbrella." The snake oil says, "I'm not a drug or a poison—I'm a food supplement; buy me." This confidence scheme is based on the specious logic that if it comes from food, it is by definition good for you. Yet we know that there are more than 2,000 naturally occurring poisons in food, and concentrating them from food to sell them as pills makes no sense at all [14]. The beans from which the starch blockers come are the source of a number of poisons, among which are substances that agglutinate red cells and that can trigger lymphocyte proliferation. These poisons are generally killed by cooking; starch blockers are usually processed uncooked bean extract.

The health food gurus sell us poison [2,10] and call it food while denouncing the safe food supply in the United States as poison. They want to get richer by selling us pills, powders, and potions instead of food, and to do this they use nutrition terrorism to make us fear the healthy food on the shelves of our grocery stores and supermarkets unless it is labeled "organic" or "natural." All food is ultimately "organic" and "natural"; all that such labeling does is raise the price. The health food industry and its snake oil promoters falsely maintain that people in the United States are dying faster than ever due to the "faulty American diet." However, the fact is that they are living longer than ever, particularly in the last 30 years and the last decade [15]. The decline continued in 1979, the last year with figures available in the

Department of Health and Human Services report titled *Health: United States, 1982* (except for increased deaths in the 15–24 age group due to automobile accidents, murders, and suicides) [16].

Food Additives

I now turn to the so-called badditives—additives in our diet. It is part of the catechism of promotion of nutrition fraud to our young to falsely inform them that they can't trust the American food supply, so they should buy expensive "health" foods. The litany falsely claims, "You can't trust nutrition scientists, so listen to us and buy what we promote." Part of this litany is the false representation that additives are bad for you, whereas, in fact, additives that are harmful are forbidden by U.S. law to be added to food. The facts regarding food additives are that sugar, salt, and corn sweeteners account for 93 percent by weight of all food additives consumed in the United States; another 6 percent is limited to 32 common substances, such as yeast, baking soda, vegetable colors, mustard, and pepper. The remaining commonly used additives are primarily flavoring substances and total only 0.07 ounce of each additive per person per year [17].

The report entitled *Diet, Nutrition and Cancer*, released in June, 1982, by the National Academy of Sciences [18], reviewed the literature on food additives and came to the conclusion that "the evidence reviewed by the Committee does not suggest that the increasing use of food additives has contributed significantly to the overall risk of cancer for humans." They concluded that there was inadequate evidence to recommend dietary changes, and they recommended as "interim guidelines" that if we changed to a more vegetarian diet with less fat in it, there might be less cancer in the United States, basing their recommendation on an inappropriate analogy to the situation with respect to cancer and smoking 20 years ago. The analogy is inappropriate because 20 years ago we knew from the work of Oscar Auerbach with beagles that smoking could generate lesions in the beagle dog. No strong similar evidence exists for the "interim guidelines"—indeed, we do not know whether following these guidelines nationally in the United States would do more good or more harm in terms of total population health. It would be more sensible if they had said, "We recommend that overweight Americans cut down to a diet with 30–35 percent of calories from fat instead of 42 percent of calories from fat because we want to help them lose weight and fat is more calorie-dense than carbohydrate and protein" [13].

Interestingly, the Russians, according to the Central Intelligence Agency (CIA) [19], have a diet much higher in grains and potatoes and much lower in fish and meat than ours. The CIA study, delivered to the Joint Economic Committees of Congress on December 1, 1982, by Henry Rowen, chairperson of the National Intelligence Council of the CIA, indicated that the average Russian consumes 3,300 calories per day, as compared with 3,500 calories per day for the average American, with 44% as grains, cereals, and potatoes (26% for Americans), 8% as meat and fish (21% for Americans), 17% as fats and oils (18% for Americans), 11% as dairy products and eggs (12% for Americans), 13% as sugar (17% for Americans), and 7% as other foods (6% for Americans). (I suspect these data refer to "calorie disappearance" rather than to actual consumption.)

Food Supplements

"Food supplement" is a term of legal art. Basically it describes things which can, at least theoretically, be extracted from food and which are sold as pills, powders, and potions to be eaten—none of which we need but which make a lot of money for their sellers. If the health food promoter can call his product a "food supplement" instead of a drug, he can sell anything, no matter how useless or dangerous. This is true of a wide variety of toxic substances [10], as well as of things not generally recognized as toxic, such as vitamins and minerals, which in large doses are toxic. The promoters of nutrition misinformation tell you that under emotional stress, your need for nutrients is increased above what your food supplies. This is untrue. An increasing number of major pharmaceutical manufacturers have been using this tactic. One company misleadingly asserts that if you drink, smoke, diet, or happen to be sick you may be "robbing your body of vitamins." Another manufacturer misleadingly warns that "stress can deplete your body of water-soluble vitamins, and daily replacement is necessary." Another plugs its unneeded products to fill the alleged "special needs of athletes." While it is true that the need for vitamins may rise slightly under physical (but not emotional) stress and in certain disease, the average American, stressed or not, is simply not in danger of vitamin deficiency. The increased needs referred to in the advertisements are in fact so trivial that they are met by almost any diet. A person who is really in danger of deficiency as a result of illness needs medical care, not vitamin pills, but these promotions are aimed at well-nourished members of the general public.

Have you ever wondered why devotees of "health food" who buy all their food from health food stores feel the need to take pills, powders, and potions as supplements on top of their healthy diet? They are willing victims of snake oil nutrition claims. Snake oil nutrition rests largely on deception by omission. For example, we see full-page advertisements saying, "Are you a vitamin underachiever? Do you smoke? Did you know that if you smoke, your blood vitamin C level is lower than if you don't smoke? Maybe you need a supplement." This is deception by omission—the *data* are omitted. If you look up the cited paper, which is Pelletier's paper on vitamin C levels of smokers as compared with nonsmokers, you do indeed find that the advertisements are true. If you don't smoke, your mean vitamin C level is 23; if you do smoke, it is 19 [20]. However, the level you need is only above 2! So if you smoke, your vitamin C level drops from 11.5 times the level you need to 9.5 times the level you need. This is deception by omission—the advertisements tell you that if you smoke, your blood vitamin C level is lower than if you don't smoke, but they don't tell you that it is still 9.5 times the level you need. Interestingly, there is a 1978 study that suggests that if you take vitamin C supplements, they may cause you to smoke more [20a]!

Young people are falsely told that they all need vitamin pills or health foods or both. Recent surveys indicate that 55 percent of all Americans are taking a vitamin, mineral, or vitamin/mineral supplement each day [21]—and this in the face of the fact that few need any of the contents and that many of the contents are not needed by anybody. For example, nobody needs biotin in a pill, because our intestinal bacteria make all we need [22], but Hoffmann-LaRoche, vitamin wholesaler to the world, has full-page advertisements in *Prevention* and other magazines asking, "Are you getting your biotin?" apparently to pressure people into demanding biotin in pills. The only way you can get biotin deficiency is by losing the lower half of your bowel containing the bacteria that make biotin, or by eating a dozen or more raw egg whites a day, since these contain avidin, which makes biotin unabsorbable [22]. Promoters misrepresent the Recommended Dietary Allowance (RDA) [23], saying that biotin is needed in the diet. But that is not true, since your bacteria make all you need. The Committee on the Uses of the RDA (Food and Nutrition Board of the National Academy of Sciences) hopefully will inform the public about these misleading uses of the RDA when their report comes out indicating the appropriate and inappropriate uses of the RDA.

Constant promotion to the public obscures adverse facts. In the *New England Journal of Medicine* [24] we recently reported that 14 of the most popular multivitamin/mineral supplements may contain from 10 to 30 percent warped and damaged vitamin B_{12} molecules, which may have been damaged by the vitamin C, or iron in the preparation, or both. These other nutrients, when concentrated, have been known since the early 1950s to warp and damage vitamin B_{12}, converting it, among other things, to various stable yellow corrinoids. We do not know whether these warped or damaged molecules are in any way harmful. Interestingly, the best-selling spirulina "B_{12}" was 80 percent analogues [25]. We are now extracting some of these analogues by high-pressure liquid chromatography and separating them out, and we are planning to feed them to human normal and malignant cells and see what they do. Perhaps some of them may kill cancer cells or normal cells, or both. Kondo and colleagues reported that two of the analogues extracted from the most popular multivitamin pill in the United States block B_{12} metabolism in mammalian cells in the test tube [26]; we do not know yet if humans absorb these particular analogues from these particular vitamin pills.

For a number of years after we first published on the subject of damage to B_{12} by vitamin C, we were attacked by people who received funds from Hoffman-LaRoche, usually not noting such funding in their publications. They claimed that our studies were invalid because when they added cyanide in the test tube, they found (as was known since 1949) that it protected B_{12} against destruction by vitamin C. We pointed out that eating cyanide has its own problems [2,24]. They also published some studies using the United States Pharmacopeia (USP) standard microbiologic assay method for measuring vitamin B_{12}, which seemed to show that B_{12} was not damaged by C. Our studies suggest that assay does not differentiate between intact B_{12} molecules and a variety of analogues because *Lactobacillus leichmannii*, the microorganism used in the USP assay, appears to grow on some analogues [24,25].

There are a wide variety of food supplements on the market that can be harmful, ranging from aloe to ginseng to yarrow, all of which contain small amounts of potentially dangerous substances [10,27]. I recently saw a young man whose girlfriend was giving him ginseng because it was supposed to have a sexually stimulating effect. What he got was the estrogen effect [10,27] and a painful gynecomastia which brought him into the hospital.

Some food supplement pills are pure frauds, such as superoxide dismutase (SOD) and RNA. Both these products are digested in the intestine, but they are falsely represented as being absorbed and effective for a wide range of miraculous purposes like preventing cancer and keeping one young forever. These are more examples of deception by omission—the promoters tell us what our own SOD and our own RNA made in our cells in species-specific human-active form can do, and neglect to tell us that the SOD and RNA pills they are selling us are not human species, are not absorbed intact, and are not worthwhile for any purpose but making money. If the yeast and sardine RNA pills sold to a gullible public actually worked, they would turn people into a young yeast or a young sardine, because RNA is a specific genetic blueprint and can only reproduce its own species. It is like the negative of a photograph; a negative of a sardine could only produce a positive with fins and scales. In a recent Postal Service action against a major RNA pill seller, defense expert witness Dr. Robert Atkins [10] produced no photographs of patients with their new fins and tails to buttress his contention that RNA pills work. Nutrition scientists know that if you eat an enzyme (such as SOD) you are not going to absorb it, because all enzymes are proteins and all proteins are digested in the intestine. Once it is digested, it is no longer SOD. So what gets absorbed is the resulting amino acids and not SOD.

Some young people swallow pure frauds as willingly as they do potentially toxic megadoses of vitamin A. All one has to do is say that something is "unorthodox" or "unconventional" or "the establishment is against it," and many of them will swallow any pill, potion, or powder. A major wholesaler represents through their Vitamin Nutrition Information Service to health professionals that doses of vitamin A up to 100,000 international units (IU) are safe [28]. In a 1982 editorial, we pointed out that cases of poisoning have occurred from just one health food store capsule of vitamin A daily, because these capsules of vitamin A usually each contain 500 percent (i.e., 25,000 IU) of the RDA. An interesting thing about the cases reported from our V.A. hospitals in 1982 is that the men with liver damage from one 25,000-IU daily capsule of vitamin A were health food faddists whose diets were largely vegetarian and therefore loaded with vitamin A; the last thing they needed was an additional 500 percent of the RDA superimposed on their diets [29]. The people to whom these pills are directed, the health food store devotees, are usually taking diets already loaded with vitamin A, which is luxus in the U.S. diet [29].

A vegetarian diet is a good way to lose weight; such diets are so high in bulk and so low in calories that it is difficult to become overweight. Strict vegetarian diets have to be modified by the addition of animal protein, or vitamin B_{12} deficiency will result; and if the diet is very high in fiber, like the Pritikin program, iron deficiency will probably occur because the iron is going to come out in the stool instead of being absorbed [30]. For example, spinach iron is only 1.5 percent absorbable. If you take the simple approach of looking at tables of metal content of foods, you will see that spinach has a reasonably high iron content, but you will not learn that spinach iron is only 1.5 percent absorbable—only one-tenth as absorbable as meat iron. You can learn this from the RDA [23] or a responsible textbook on nutrition [22], but not from food tables.

An interesting thing about one of the two vegetarian patients who got liver toxicity from taking one health food capsule of vitamin A a day is that one could not make the diagnosis from the serum vitamin A level, since it was not elevated. This vegetarian had protein undernutrition and could not make adequate nutrient carrier proteins, so his serum vitamin A level was actually low even though his liver was loaded with vitamin A and he had severe liver damage. Another factor may have been involved, because once a person gets liver damage, his ability to make serum protein falls; so this patient may have started off with a high serum vitamin A level from the 25,000-IU capsule on top of his vegetarian diet. Then, as the excess vitamin A deposited in his liver and progressively damaged it, his liver became progressively unable to make carrier proteins adequately, especially with his vegetarian diet, thus probably producing inadequacy of one of the essential amino acids [31].

Summary and Conclusions

This chapter has reflected on just a few of the harms resulting from fad diets and from the false allegations that you can't trust the U.S. diet, that additives are badditives, and that everybody needs food supplements because nobody eats a balanced diet. Nutrition nonsense is accepted because we have not learned how to think; we have not learned to ask, "How do I know the things that I know?" We do not ask, "Is it better than doing nothing? Is it safer than doing nothing?"

Young people often believe the false claims of nutrition cultism as expounded in irresponsible magazines. For instance, an article entitled "Advice on Supplements" in *Family Circle* (October 5, 1982, p. 147) says: "More experts agree: We need vitamin and/or mineral supplements. The reason? Most of us don't eat a balanced diet and much of the food we do eat has been processed in some way—and valuable vitamins and minerals are lost in processing. The real problem arises when you try to determine which vitamins you should take and how you should take them."

The truth is that most of us get all the vitamins and minerals we need in our daily food. In one study, 67 percent of patients used nutritional supplements on a daily basis or had used them to "treat" an illness; 80 percent believed the false claim that supplements increased energy, vitality, and physical strength [32]. Supplements can produce many harms [2,10,33].

It is untrue that most of us do not eat a balanced diet. All a balanced diet means is that you eat from each of the four basic food groups—when you look back at the end of the day, you have had four portions from the grain group (which includes breads and cereals—and white bread gives you better protein than whole wheat, as noted in the September 1982 *Consumer Reports*); four portions from the fruit, vegetable, and fruit juice group, including at least one that is fresh and uncooked; two portions from the milk and milk products group, including cheese, yogurt, and even ice cream; and two portions from the meat group, which includes poultry, fish, nuts, and some dry beans (because the lead nutrient in the meat group is protein and these products are all high in protein, although the protein in nuts and dry beans is not animal protein and therefore not quite as good as the protein in animal products; nuts and beans are also devoid of vitamin B_{12}). This adds up to 1,200 calories, so the "basic four" is a sound diet for weight loss, and beyond that we can eat anything we want—including the fifth food group designated by the Department of Agriculture: fats, oils, sugar, and alcohol (in moderation and variety, of course)—to get the calories to sustain our weight.

Thus one can see that much of the cultist catechism that "junk foods" are bad for you is simple nonsense—junk foods come from the four food groups and are good for you in moderation, like all food. It is bad nutrition to violate the basic rules of sound nutrition, which are moderation and variety. Thus, a diet consisting exclusively of pizza, or of hot dogs, or of hamburgers is bad nutrition, but each of these foods is good nutrition. A cheeseburger with lettuce and tomato, for example, includes all of the four food groups—the bun is the grain group, the lettuce and tomato are the fruit and vegetable group, and both the grain and fruit and vegetable groups are rich in fiber; the burger and the cheese are rich in animal protein and vitamin B_{12}; and the burger is also rich in highly absorbable minerals—the iron in meat is absorbed five times as well as the iron in vegetables. The statement that "much of the food we eat has been processed in some way—and valuable vitamins and minerals are lost in processing" is misleading because the fact is that processing—in the factory or in the home—generally means heating, and while heating does destroy a variable amount of some vitamins, the amount left is adequate as part of a balanced diet (which simply means a diet containing moderate amounts of a variety of foods). Minerals are not destroyed by heat, although some are removed to a variable degree when foods are finely particulate and cooked in water, which can wash out some of the minerals into the water. Again, this is no problem in the context of a balanced diet, which most of us get. In fact, measurements of vitamins and minerals in blood and living tissue of most Americans yields normal levels.

Food consumption surveys which show that some people are getting only 60 percent of the RDA of vitamin B_6 or some other vitamin do not mean that those people are not getting enough of that vitamin. The RDAs are deliberately set at levels not only to encompass the range of daily need of Americans, but to allow enough extra so that there is storage of a substantial reserve in tissues; thus, if by some unlikely possibility, days or weeks go by when a person does not eat a particular vitamin or mineral or does not absorb it because of some intestinal upset, the body can draw on its own stored nutrients [23]. Contrary to the false claims of those who make money promoting the sale of unnecessary vitamin supplements (which do nothing for us except give us expensive urine), a percentage of the water-soluble vitamins we get is in fact stored. For example, the RDA for vitamin C of 60 mg per day causes the storage in the liver and other tissues of enough vitamin C to last for 150 days if we eat no vitamin C at all for that period of time. In general, we have stored from our food sufficiently large quantities of each of the water-soluble vitamins in our tissues so that most of the additional water-soluble vitamins we take in a pill are urinated out.

The basic four food groups remain the basis of sound nutrition [2,10,22, 23]. The three words *balance*, *variety*, and *moderation* remain the keystones of nutrition science as applied to what we eat. Variety, of course, means the variety not only of four food groups, but also *within* each group. This is of crucial importance. Balance means not only a balance of foods, but also of calories consumed in relation to calories burned.

References

1. Morowitz, H.J. Drinking hemlock and other nutritional matters. *Hosp. Pract.* 13:155, 1978.

2. Herbert, V. *Nutrition Cultism*, 3rd rev. ed. Philadelphia: George F. Stickley, 1981.

3. Fiske, E.B. Low reading comprehension found. *New York Times*, November 12, 1981, p. 13.

4. Katz, J.C. Science—The missing link in general education; scientific literacy is national news. *Columbia College Today* 8:19–20, 1981.

5. Nobel laureate says scientists must forcefully reject cult attacks. *Peninsula Times Tribune* (Oakland, Calif.), March 19, 1981, pp. 13–15.

6. Herbert, V. Will questionable nutrition overwhelm nutrition science? *Am. J. Clin. Nutr.* 34:2848–2853, 1981.

7. Bo-Linn, G.W., Santa Ana, C.A., Morawski, S.O., Fordtran, J.S. Starch blockers: Their effect on calorie absorption from a high-starch meal. *N. Engl. J. Med.* 307:1413–1416, 1982.

8. Rosenberg, I.H. Starch blockers: Still no calorie-free lunch. *N. Engl. J. Med.* 307:1444–1445, 1982.

9. Stein, J., Urdang, L. *The Random House Dictionary of the English Language* (unabridged edition). New York: Random House, 1967. Pp. 1017, 1536.

10. Herbert, V., Barrett, S. *Vitamins and 'Health' Foods: The Great American Hustle*. Philadelphia: George F. Stickley, 1981.

11. Hambidge, K.M. Hair analyses—Worthless for vitamins, limited for minerals. *Am. J. Clin. Nutr.* 36:943–949, 1982.

12. Calcium supplements with a touch of lead. *Consumer Reports*, vol. 47, no. 9, 1982, pp. 478–479.

13. Herbert, V. Nutrition. In *Medical Update 1983*. Chicago: World Book, 1982. Pp. 222–224.

14. Committee on Food Protection, Food and Nutrition Board of the National Research Council. *Toxicants Occurring Naturally in Foods*, 2nd ed. Washington, D.C.: National Academy of Sciences, 1973.

15. McGinniss, J.M. Recent health gains for adults. *N. Engl. J. Med.* 306:617–673, 1982.

16. Death rates decline for all except young people. *New York Times*, January 9, 1983, p. 21.

17. Committee on Diet, Nutrition and Cancer, Assembly of Life Sciences of the National Research Council. *Diet, Nutrition and Cancer*. Washington, D.C.: National Academy Press, 1982.

18. Block, Z. *It's All on the Label: Understanding Food, Additives and Nutrition*. Boston: Little, Brown, 1981.

19. Soviet diet standbys: Cereals and potatoes. *New York Times*, January 14, 1983, p. 16.

20. Pelletier, O. Vitamin C and cigarette smokers. *Ann. N.Y. Acad. Sci.* 258:156–168, 1975.

20a. Schachter, S. Pharmacological and psychological determinants of smoking. *Ann. Intern. Med.* 88:104–114, 1978.

21. Schutz, H.G., Read, M., Bendel, R., et al. Food supplement usage in seven western states. *Am. J. Clin. Nutr.* 36:897–902, 1982.

22. Goodhart, R.S., Shils, M.E. (Eds.), *Modern Nutrition in Health and Disease*, 6th ed. Philadelphia: Lea and Febiger, 1980.

23. Committee on Dietary Allowances, Food and Nutrition Board of the National Research Council. *Recommended Dietary Allowances*, 9th ed. Washington, D.C.: National Academy of Sciences, 1980.

24. Herbert, V., Drivas, G., Foscaldi, R., et al. Multivitamin/mineral food supplements containing vitamin B_{12} may also contain analogues of vitamin B_{12}. *N. Engl. J. Med.* 307:255–256, 1982.

25. Herbert, V., Drivas, G. Spirulina and vitamin B_{12}. *J.A.M.A.* 248:3096–3097, 1982.

26. Kondo, H., Binder, M.J., Kolhouse, J.F., et al. Presence and formation of cobalamin analogues in multivitamin/minerals pills. *J. Clin. Invest.* 70:889–898, 1982.

27. Tyler, V.E. *The Honest Herbal.* Philadelphia: George F. Stickley, 1982.

28. Vitamin Nutrition Information Service, Hoffmann-LaRoche. Vitamin safety: A factual perspective. *Vitamin Issues* 2:1–5, 1981.

29. Herbert, V. Toxicity of 25,000 IU vitamin A supplements in 'health' food users. *Am. J. Clin. Nutr.* 36:185–186, 1982.

30. The Pritikin program: Claims vs. facts. *Consumer Reports*, vol. 47, no. 10, 1982, pp. 513–518.

31. Hatoff, D.E., Gertler, S.L., Miyai, K., et al. Hypervitaminosis A unmasked by acute viral hepatitis. *Gastroenterology* 82:124–128, 1982.

32. English, E.C., Carl, J.W. Use of nutritional supplements by family practice patients. *J.A.M.A.* 246:2719–2721, 1981.

33. Marshall, C. *Vitamins and Minerals: Help or Harm?* Philadelphia: George F. Stickley, 1983.

Discussion

Questions were addressed to the panel of speakers, which consisted of Dr. Alfin-Slater, Dr. Hegarty, and Dr. Herbert.

Topics of dietary modification, particularly the issues of weight control and meeting basic needs for vitamins and minerals, aroused the greatest interest. The audience was cautioned against the use of any diet that has an energy content of less than 800 calories. Such a diet cannot be nutritionally adequate; that is, it cannot satisfy all basic nutritional requirements. At best, diets such as the Cambridge diet, when they are indicated, can be regarded only as a supplement to a regular diet.

The panel did not suggest elimination of specific foods from a diet for purposes of weight loss; rather, they argued that caloric restriction combined with some exercise would serve this purpose. For example, sugar per se is not bad in that it is pure carbohydrate; the danger of certain sugars is that when present in certain "sticky" foods they may remain in the mouth to be digested by bacteria, which causes formation of substances that are erosive to dental enamel.

The presence of fiber—or bulk, as it used to be called—in the diet is generally regarded as beneficial. It provides for the increased entry of water into the colon and thereby helps to prevent constipation. Fiber is thought to aid in preventing colon cancer by decreasing colonic transit time and increasing the turnover of intestinal flora. Conversely, excess dietary fiber is undesirable because it binds trace minerals and makes them unavailable to the body.

There are specific indications for supplementation of the normal diet with some vitamins and minerals. This issue was also considered by previous panelists. The average American diet has a marginal iron content. Supplemental iron is indicated for children from birth to about 5 years of age, at the onset of puberty, and for women during the child-bearing years, especially those on vegetarian diets. Some suggested that the elderly may benefit from dietary vitamin supplementation, since their absorption of nutrients is not as complete as in younger people. Dr. Herbert disagreed with this view, citing published reports in support [1]. However, the elderly frequently undergo drug therapy, which may profoundly influence the absorption and effectiveness of, and therefore increase the requirement for, dietary vitamins and trace minerals.

The need for dietary calcium supplementation is debatable except during pregnancy and lactation. Echoing Dr. DeLuca's earlier remarks, the panel agreed that dietary calcium intake is normally sufficient. If calcium intake is decreased before age 50, then the likelihood of osteoporosis past age 50 is much less. Dietary calcium is at least as important during the years of bone formation as it is later on, since during the earlier years calcium (especially when paired with exercise) increases bone density, whereas during the later years adequate dietary calcium intake lessens calcium resorption from bone. Dietary supplements of vitamin D are usually not indicated for the elderly.

The scientific basis for the use of herbs (as food additives) was questioned. The panel pointed out that the use of herbs is based on folklore. As a group, herbs represent many different classes of substances that have widely varying activities. Herbs may be flavoring agents, medicants, toxins, or carcinogens. Therefore, the recommendation was made to seek out specific information from reputable, published sources.

A lengthy debate ensued concerning the question of protein-energy malnutrition. This is a problem that affects particularly children, but it occurs less frequently in the United States than in some of the developing nations. A consensus emerged on several points that apply to nutrition in general. Prolonged breast feeding prevents protein-energy malnutrition. However, milk is poor in iron and copper, which may result in a deficiency even though breast milk iron is exceptionally well absorbed. The consequences are relatively mild and can be dealt with on a separate basis.

Protein-energy malnutrition is a broad problem that has to be solved on an international scale. Experience has taught that food shortages have to be remedied with foods that are familiar to the recipients. Thus, simple redistribution of excess food is a well-meaning but naive approach. Furthermore, public health and sanitation programs must accompany the availability of food. Thus, the problem of protein-energy malnutrition requires decisions on a global scale that must be made not only by nutritionists but also by politicians, economists, planners, and educators.

In the United States, nutrition education has become more prominent than before. Both reputable and disreputable publications on the topic of nutrition are appearing in greater numbers, and many new associations, both responsible and irresponsible, concern themselves with nutritional science and education. The American Dietetic Association has established criteria for the accreditation of coordinated undergraduate programs leading to the baccalaureate degree and for postbaccalaureate internships in dietetics. Furthermore, many continuing education programs are available to health care personnel at all levels, and approximately one-fourth of all medical schools in the United States are now offering formal courses in nutrition to their students. For the layman, the problem exists of discerning nutritionally responsible from irresponsible information. Several reliable, factual sources were suggested: *Health Quackery* is a book published in 1980 by Consumers Union, who also publish a monthly column in their periodical *Consumer Reports*; in addition, the Food and Drug Administration publishes a monthly magazine, *FDA Consumer*, which is available by subscription.

Reference

1. Willmore, D.W. Parenteral nutrition in burn patients. In Greep, J.M., et al. (Eds.), *Current Concepts in Parenteral Nutrition.* The Hague: Nijhoff Medical Division, 1977. Pp. 227–239.

IV Nutrition in the Elderly

11 Aging and Factors Influencing the Nutritional Status of the Elderly

Clifford F. Gastineau, M.D., Ph.D.

Growing older is a very personal matter. We sense the signs of aging in ourselves and in others, but rarely do we examine these signs in detail or articulate our reactions to their significance. Thinking about the processes of aging reminds us of the inevitability of the cessation of life, and while it may not be possible for us to comprehend fully the prospect of our own death, we are led to wonder what will be the consequences of aging to us as individuals.

External Manifestations of Age

In our years of childhood and adolescence, we see ourselves growing both in size and in the functional capacity of our bodies, while we see in older people the merging of the stages of maturity and of advancing age. Changes in the skin include thinning with a transparency that reveals clearly the pattern of superficial veins and is similar to that seen in the atrophy of skin characteristic of protein-calorie malnutrition or Cushing's syndrome. Other dermal changes that we all recognize as characteristic of aging are laxness with wrinkling, irregular pigmentation, ectasia of superficial blood vessels, and areas of scaling called actinic keratoses which tend to undergo malignant change. Many of these dermal changes are accelerated by exposure to sunlight, especially in people of Celtic origin, so much so that a person who cultivates a deep suntan can be regarded as trying to hasten the aging of his skin. Scalp hair is thinned and loses pigment irregularly, the nose and ears progressively enlarge, the gait is less confident, and the distribution of body fat is changed. Body fat tends to become less centrifugal and more centripetal, as well as less subcutaneous and more visceral [1]. While subcutaneous fat is relatively more prominent in the face, neck, and extremities than about the trunk in youth, the proportion is reversed as age advances. The amount of fat around the kidneys and within the abdominal cavity in the omentum becomes greater with aging, while subcutaneous fat tends to diminish in proportion. Parenthetically, it might be said that measurements of skinfold thickness will not accurately reflect the state of adipose reserves unless appropriate allowances are made for age. The skinfold tables by Durnin permit such calculations [1].

Loss of stature is another characteristic of aging. It is primarily a consequence of thinning of intervertebral disks, a decrease in the vertical dimensions of vertebral bodies, and an increasing kyphosis [2].

Mechanisms of Aging

While we are all aware of these external changes of aging, the mechanisms by which we age are less obvious. There are many theories of aging, no one of which appears to explain all aspects of the process.

The Cell

We can focus our attention first on the cell and the fundamental experiments of Hayflick [3,4], which show that cultured cells have a limited life span. Fibroblasts from normal human embryos will survive about 50 serial subcultivations or population doublings, while fibroblasts derived from older people have a proportionately shorter survival time. It is proposed that functional decrements which precede the loss of capacity for cell division are responsible for aging and the death of the individual before cell division ceases. It is thought that the "clock" which limits the life span of a cell line is located in the nucleus. Cell life expectancy is reduced in cells derived from individuals having diabetes, progeria, and Werner's syndrome [5].

Genetic Factors

How is the life span of the cell determined? Genetic factors do determine the life spans of various species. Man is one of the longer-lived species, and some families do seem to have an unusually high proportion of elderly persons. It is possible that a limited number of genes may carry the propensity for long life, but another explanation is that our genetic equipment may confer greater or lesser life expectancy through multiple mechanisms which render us vulnerable or resistant to various disease processes. A "longevity homeostasis gene complex which includes genes linked to immune response loci and genes that control endocrine balance" has been postulated as the mechanism that determines optimal longevity [6].

Immunologic Competence

Progressive loss of immunologic competence with aging may result in increased frequency of diseases that involve autoimmune mechanisms, such as maturity onset diabetes, neoplasia, and various connective tissue disorders. Loss of immune competence with aging has been identified in both humoral and cell-mediated systems.

Mutagenicity

Random errors in cell replication with accumulation of abnormal gene products may gradually lead to decreased functional capacity and finally to extinction of a cell line. These processes can occur simply as chance affairs or as the result of mutagenic environmental influences. Longevity may be a consequence of increased ability of the cell to metabolize and dispose of carcinogens or mutagenic substances [7]. Ionizing radiation is another source of mutagenic forces. Free radicals arise from abnormal, uncontrolled chemical reactions occurring within cells that may be provoked by certain spontaneously occurring processes or by exposure to ionizing radiation, ultraviolet light, or toxic substances known as initiators [8]. Molecules within cell membranes (particularly lipids) and other cell components such as nucleic acids are very susceptible to damage by free radicals. Chemical carcinogenesis and radiation pathology may occur through such mechanisms—and aging itself may be speeded by the cumulative effects of both endogenous and environmental factors. Antioxidants such as vitamins C and E and selenium-glutathione peroxidase provide some degree of protection against lipid peroxidation and other free radical pathology. One could also propose that some of the food additives used for their antioxidation properties might be equally effective in this role—perhaps even more so because their water-soluble character may permit better diffusion of the substance into cells.

Membrane Receptors

Membrane receptors for a number of hormones have been found to decrease by 50 to 75 percent with age, although binding affinity does not seem to change [9]. In contrast, the activities of cellular enzymes do not seem to change with age, although the decreased capacity of liver microsomal enzymes to metabolize drugs seems to constitute an exception to this generalization [10].

Environmental Factors

Among environmental forces, dietary factors have been found to have a substantial effect in influencing life span [11] and are implicated in human longevity. In cold-blooded animals, lowering of the metabolic rate by exposure to cold will extend the life span, but in warm-blooded animals this is scarcely feasible. In homoiotherms the most effective means of extending life is dietary restriction begun soon after weaning. If underfeeding is delayed until after growth has been completed, life span may be either prolonged or shortened depending on the composition of the diet; if underfeeding is imposed during the suckling period, the life may be shortened. To what extent the results of animal experiments can be applied to human nutrition is uncertain. Animals subjected to chronic underfeeding may be able to survive and exhibit their greater potential for longevity in a protected laboratory environment, but they may be vulnerable to bacterial and parasitic diseases and at a competitive disadvantage because of decreased strength and endurance in natural, free-living conditions. In one series of experiments [11], self-selected diets were effective in maintaining health during the first half of life but increased susceptibility to diseases of later life.

Nutrition in Older Age

Two questions about human nutrition come to mind: Is there a particular diet that will favor maximal longevity within our genetic potential? Are the nutritional requirements of the elderly different from those of persons who have reached their maturity? With respect to the first question, I would venture the opinion that there is a rather wide range of composition and quantity of diet compatible with a good life span. Humans are not rats, nor is humanity a rat colony. Generalizations from the effects of diet on longevity in animals, based for the most part on studies using rats, cannot be applied directly to humans. Furthermore, the human race is much more diverse genetically than is a rat colony, and nutritional strategies that might favor long life in one individual might have an adverse or null effect in another. The person genetically disposed to hypertension might be benefited by a diet restricted in sodium and limited in calories to provide distinct leanness. Another individual less vulnerable to hypertension might be able to enjoy salt-rich foods (and in some societies at times in history, preservation of some foods with salt was ensurance that there would be any food at all at certain seasons of the year). The obese person not vulnerable to diseases such as diabetes or hypertension would perhaps have a greater capacity to survive serious illnesses and injuries by virtue of a more generous reserve of calories in the form of adipose tissue. Thus, a general plan of dietary advice is difficult to devise with any confidence, as evidenced by the recent debates about dietary goals. With respect to the individual, however, one could argue that people having relatives with hypertension, or any trend in that direction themselves, should systematically restrict sodium intake; those with relatives who have died in early or middle life of stroke or of myocardial infarct, or who have increased serum lipids themselves, should restrict dietary fats in the fashion most effective in controlling serum lipid levels; and those with relatives having diabetes should avoid thiazide diuretics and cortisone analogues. All these groups might seek to achieve and maintain a distinctly lean weight, perhaps with about 15 percent or less of body weight as fat. Unfortunately, there is little information regarding the extent to which achieving distinct leanness measured in precise terms of body composition may lessen the risk of these diseases.

The second question, whether the nutrient requirements of the elderly differ from those of individuals in their early and middle mature years, is also not easily answered. The widespread tendency for people to take dietary supplements of vitamins, minerals, and substances of unverified efficacy is commonly exploited and is today big business. There is little evidence that the need for vitamins or minerals is increased in older age [12], although the issue is still a matter worthy of further investigation. There is, however, a body of evidence that protein requirements are increased in older age [13], perhaps to a level greater than the 0.8 g per kg specified in the Recommended Dietary Allowances. No physiologic mechanism comes to mind, however, to explain a qualitative difference in protein need among the elderly [12]. Perhaps as a practical matter the question of whether the elderly require a diet of greater nutrient density because of their age does not require a definite answer. The elderly are more often ill or injured and hence experience recurring periods of stress-induced protein depletion. Periods of needed repletion are required with greater frequency, and hence one can argue that the elderly should take care to observe conventional rules for obtaining adequate nutrition but that there is no need for special diets or dietary supplements.

Calorie requirements do decrease steadily with age, and if the calorie consumption practiced in young adult life is continued in later life, obesity will result.

Decrements in Physiologic Functions with Age

Homeostatic Capacity

Aging is associated with a steady decrease of most functions [4,14] in a linear fashion at a rate of 0.8 to 0.9 percent per year past the age of 30. There is thus a resulting decrease in homeostatic capacity. The failing ability to adapt to nearly all stresses is reflected in a greater morbidity, prolonged convalescence, and a greater chance of death with all illnesses and injuries. With advancing age even minor illnesses may prove lethal. Decrements in function and hence adaptive capacity with aging are greater for performances that require the integrated activity of a number of organ systems than for those involving a single system [14].

Drug Effects

With decreasing renal function and impaired capacity for hepatic disposal of drugs, the elderly person is more vulnerable to drug reactions and intoxications [10]. Drugs can impair appetite and taste and in this manner lead to impaired nutrition. Certain drugs such as digoxin can lead directly to anorexia, while drugs that have anticholinergic properties may impair eating through inhibition of salivary secretion. Many of the antidepressant drugs share in this property, and one may not suspect them of being responsible for contributing to impairment of nutritional status. On the other hand, some antidepressants may increase appetite and cause weight gain.

The increased frequency of illness among the elderly increases the likelihood of multiple medications. The elderly are susceptible to the claims of advertisers for many over-the-counter drugs. They also tend to use nutritional supplements, which may have some adverse effects on appetite. Furthermore, the elderly person may unwittingly invite excessive prescribing of medications by visiting a physician to fulfill social needs. The lonely elderly person may seek some solace by a visit to the physician—it is a socially approved way of having a visit with someone and has the additional virtue of casting the individual in a role that occupies center stage. In order to justify such a visit, however, a symptom must be produced and discussed at the time of the visit. The symptom may or may not have much relevance to the individual's actual state of health, but to complete the scenario and give justification for the visit the physician then must carry out some therapeutic act. Most commonly this act will consist of the writing out of a prescription for a drug which will yield some relief of symptoms. Unfortunately, this way of dealing with the patient's expressed concern may produce an unnecessary and undesirable proliferation of medicines. Particularly if a patient visits a number of physicians, he may accumulate a remarkable list of medications with a complex schedule of administration. Some of these drugs may interact with others and produce ill effects. Often an equally satisfactory outcome in satisfying a patient's desires can be accomplished by reviewing the entire list of medications he is taking, including those not prescribed by a physician, and perhaps simplifying and revising the schedule while eliminating those drugs that have no clear therapeutic benefit.

Reasons for Limitation of Food Choice and Consumption by the Elderly

Food choices may become limited for economic reasons. Facilities for food preparation for the person living alone may not permit convenient preparation of balanced meals. The elderly often become prejudiced regarding food choices for a variety of reasons. They are often preoccupied with bodily functions such as constipation, and digestive discomforts may be blamed on certain foods, thus further limiting the variety of foods accepted by the individual. Missing teeth and poorly fitted dentures interfere with chewing and favor the choice of softer foods. Poorly chewed foods, particularly meats, may add to digestive discomforts.

Dietary Restrictions

Many elderly people need restriction of dietary sodium, and this can limit both the enjoyment and the selection of foods. Inappropriate dietary restrictions also have the potential for impairing nutrition. For example, elderly persons will often eliminate eggs in an attempt to reduce the threat of atherosclerosis, although eggs may be one of the less expensive sources of iron and of high biologic quality protein, and are in a form convenient for preparation and consumption by a person living alone. Although one can argue that lessening the consumption of saturated fat and of cholesterol in early and middle life will retard atherogenesis, such dietary restrictions beyond the age of perhaps 60 years appear to yield little benefit [15]. Nevertheless, the elderly person who has experienced a stroke or myocardial infarction will naturally be apprehensive about further ischemic episodes and will obtain reassurance from adhering to a diet restricted in fat. One must be careful, however, not to casually recommend "going easy" on certain dietary selections. What is intended as a low-key modification of the diet may be interpreted by the patient in a very rigid manner.

Role of Alcohol

Alcohol can be a major contributor to malnutrition, and alcoholism may not be suspected in the elderly person. Alcohol can impair nutritional status through numerous mechanisms including calorie dilution. Alcohol is a concentrated source of nutrient-free calories and can displace a large proportion of the day's quota of food calories, thus lowering the nutrient density of the diet consumed.

On the other hand, a small amount of alcohol in the form of wine or beer in an atmosphere of socialization has been found useful in nursing homes, permitting lessened use of tranquilizers and generally favoring improved mood and activity of the elderly [16]. Alcohol is not a good nighttime sedative, however, since it disturbs the normal sleep pattern.

What Is Our Potential Life Span?

Whatever the mechanism or combination of mechanisms that are responsible for aging and thereby for limiting life span, one could attempt to estimate average life expectancy if disease could be excluded from epidemiologic data. One such estimate concludes: "Under ideal conditions, 66% of natural deaths would occur in persons 81 to 99 years of age and 95% in persons aged 77 to 93 years" [17].

Can the individual hope to achieve this potential? The answer is uncertain. Perhaps by further research and better knowledge of the forces that render us susceptible to disease, we can learn to avoid these potentially lethal sources. The diet that achieves maximal growth rates in childhood may not be the one to provide protection from the degenerative diseases which are manifest in older age but have their roots in youth. Exercise and continued activity may postpone the steady decline of some physiologic functions. Continued attention to nutritional principles while adapting our strategies to the needs of the individual perhaps offers our best hope for the moment.

Summary

Among the external manifestations of aging, dermal changes and changes in distribution of body fat are prominent. Accurate assessment of nutritional status by skinfold thickness measurements must take these changes of age into account. The mechanisms of aging are complex and varied. Factors intrinsic to the cell, genetics, immunologic competence, mutagens, cell membrane alterations, and environmental exposures all influence the aging process. The remarkable genetic diversity of humans makes it improbable that an all-inclusive dietary prescription can be made which would result in optimal longevity for all individuals. General principles of nutrition should be followed but modified as required for each individual. The decreasing calorie requirements with an increased requirement for protein as age increases should be recognized. Factors that accelerate the decline in physiologic function seen with aging, such as drug therapy and alcohol, should be recognized and minimized if possible. A healthy life-style with adequate exercise and continued activity, combined with adequate nutrition, offers the best hope for good health with advancing age.

References

1. Durnin, J.V.G.A., Wormersley, J. Body fat assessed from total body density and its estimation from skin fold thickness. *Br. J. Nutr.* 32:79–97, 1974.

2. Mitchell, C.O., Lipschitz, D.A. Detection of protein-calorie malnutrition in the elderly. *Am. J. Clin. Nutr.* 35:398-406, 1982.

3. Hayflick, L. The cell biology of human aging. *N. Engl. J. Med.* 295:1302–1308, 1976.

4. Hayflick, L. Cell biology of aging. *Fed. Proc.* 38:1847–1850, 1979.

5. Goldstein, S., Harley, C.B. In vitro studies of age associated diseases. *Fed. Proc.* 38:1862–1867, 1979.

6. Yunis, E.J., Greenbert, L.J. Immunopathology of aging. *Fed. Proc.* 33:2017–2019, 1974.

7. Schwartz, A.G., Moore, C.J. Inverse correlation between species life span and capacity of cultured fibroblasts to metabolize polycyclic hydrocarbon carcinogens. *Fed. Proc.* 38:1989–1992, 1979.

8. Demopolous, H.B. The basis of free radical pathology. *Fed. Proc.* 32:1859–1861, 1973.

9. Roth, G.S. Hormone receptor changes during adulthood and senescence; significance for aging research. *Fed. Proc.* 38:1910–1914, 1979.

10. Gillette, J.R. Biotransformation of drugs during aging. *Fed. Proc.* 38:1900–1909, 1979.

11. Ross, M.H. Dietary behavior and longevity. *Nutr. Rev.* 35:257–265, 1977.

12. Watkin, D.M. Nutrition for the aging and aged. In Goodhart, R.J., Shils, M.E. (Eds.), *Modern Nutrition in Health and Disease*, 6th ed. Philadelphia: Lea and Febiger, 1980. Pp. 781-813.

13. Gersovitz, M., Motil, K., Munro, H.N., et al. Human protein requirements: Assessment of the adequacy of current recommended dietary allowance for dietary protein in elderly men and women. *Am. J. Clin. Nutr.* 35:6–14, 1982.

14. Shock, N.W. Systems physiology and aging. *Fed. Proc.* 38:161–162, 1979.

15. Whyte, H.M. Potential effect on coronary-heart-disease morbidity of lowering the blood-cholesterol. *Lancet* 1:906, 1975.

16. Watkin, D.M. Role of alcoholic beverages in gerontology. In Gastineau, C.F., Darby, W., Turner, T. (Eds.), *Fermented Food Beverages in Nutrition*. New York: Academic Press, 1979. Pp. 226–243.

17. Fries, J.F. Aging, natural death, and the compression of morbidity. *N. Engl. J. Med.* 303:130–135, 1980.

12 How the Elderly Eat in the United States

Patricia B. Swan, Ph.D.

How do the elderly among us eat? The information available suggests that they eat very much like everyone else, only a little less. Unfortunately, however, we do not have adequate information about the food consumption or nutritional status of persons over 65 years of age. Four major cross-sectional surveys of our population [1–4] carried out within the last 15 years form the core of our knowledge about nutrition of the elderly. These are supplemented by several small surveys of specific groups of elderly persons, often those living in institutions or participating in special feeding programs. Yet the sum of this information is inadequate for the large task of separating out influential factors and drawing firm conclusions about the food intake of the elderly.

Changes in Food Intake with Age

Cross-sectional studies suggest that there are several differences between the food intake of young adults and that of old adults. There are serious limitations, however, to our ability to interpret cross-sectional studies. It is impossible to tell whether differences in the food consumption of these groups are the result of changes that occurred in the food intake of individuals over time, or if the differences result from the fact that persons with certain eating patterns have a better chance of surviving to old age and thus constitute a larger portion of the elderly. Whichever interpretation is correct, it is important for us to be able to make the distinction and to be able to use this knowledge in our health care programs.

The lack of longitudinal studies of food consumption—that is, measurements for the same individuals over time—is a serious limitation to our understanding of food intake. From a small longitudinal study of elderly women living alone, Exton-Smith [5] has suggested that elderly individuals who remain healthy and active make very little change in their food consumption over time, whereas those who develop health problems are likely to reduce their food consumption and have undesirably low nutrient intakes. Increasing numbers of the elderly in our population will doubtless encourage further investigation of apparent changes in food consumption with age.

Many generalizations have been made about nutrition of the elderly. Often they have been made in the absence of the kind of information that is required for making well-founded conclusions about factors influencing food intake. Some of these generalizations are drawn from accurate observations for certain groups of the elderly; others are inaccurate descriptions for all groups. The once popular myth that there is a "tea and toast" set among elderly women has been rather well dispelled. Overgeneralizations, however, are more difficult to correct. For example, attention to poverty among the elderly has led to a common misconception that most elderly persons live in poverty. In fact, though the proportion of individuals with very low incomes does increase after age 60, 75 to 80 percent of the elderly are not living in poverty. Poverty does influence food consumption, but it does so for all age groups.

Exton-Smith [5] has presented and examined a list of factors that affect the nutritional status of the elderly. This list includes most of the factors commonly mentioned, including ignorance or lack of education, social isolation, physical disability, mental decline, special diets, poverty, impaired appetite, problems in chewing and swallowing, malabsorption, alcoholism, drugs, and increased nutrient needs. Each one of these factors is a reality for some, but none is true for most elderly persons. Thus, in citing these factors, the danger is that they will be overgeneralized and treated as norms rather than as aberrations that appear with increased frequency in this population.

Munro [6] has emphasized the variation in nutrient needs found among the elderly. Some of these variations result from the factors listed above. However, he has also emphasized that the factors of greatest importance are habits of eating and exercise formed early in adult life. These habits provide a constant basis for practices throughout life.

Thus, factors can be identified that will tend to cause changes in food consumption and nutritional status over time, but evidence is limited as to their importance in explaining differences in food intake. An alternative explanation for observed differences in food intake with age, that individuals with certain dietary patterns (e.g., relatively low food intakes) have a greater chance for survival to old age, is an interesting possibility that needs more exploration.

Food Needs

Nutrient needs do not change greatly with age. However, there is a decline in metabolic rate with age and, in many individuals, a decline in physical activity. The observed decline in caloric intake with age is, therefore, not surprising (Table 12-1). There is little evidence that healthy individuals have

Table 12–1
Nutrient Intakes of U.S. Adults

Sex and Age (Years)	Number of Subjects Surveyed	Food Energy (kcal)[a]	Ca (mg)	Fe (mg)	Mg (mg)	Vitamin B_6 (mg)	Vitamin A (IU)	Vitamin C (mg)
Males								
23-34	770	2,449	830	16	303	1.8	5,278	95
65-74	295	1,970	729	14	287	1.6	6,834	100
75 +	127	1,808	679	13	267	1.5	6,693	96
Females								
23-34	949	1,616	604	11	217	1.2	4,335	76
65-74	377	1,444	566	11	227	1.2	6,218	92
75 +	197	1,367	591	10	214	1.2	5,931	90

Source: Nationwide Food Consumption Survey, Spring 1977 [3]. Based on 24-hour recalls.
[a]Average intake for the group.

increased nutrient needs with age, but for those individuals with impaired absorption or chronic illnesses there may be increased nutrient requirements. Certainly, acute infections or other illnesses may have a marked influence on requirements. To the extent that elderly persons experience these problems more frequently than the young, they may exhibit a wider range in their nutrient needs. Low calorie intake coupled with a stress on other nutrient needs may suggest that nutritional supplementation should be considered. There is evidence that one-fourth to one-half of the elderly take nutrition supplements [7,8], but often they are not choosing these supplements on the basis of recommendation by a physician. This rate of supplement use, however, may not be very different from that found for younger adults. Recognition that many elderly persons use nutrition supplements presents an opportunity to the physician to talk about supplementation with elderly patients and to make helpful recommendations about whether or not to use supplements and, if so, which ones. These recommendations are probably best made on an individual basis due to variation in elderly patients [5]. The use of nutrition supplements should not be construed as lessening the need to pay attention to food intake.

Food has many values other than as a source of nutrients. Its psychological and sociological importance for people of all ages is unquestioned. It may be that these aspects of food intake are especially important to the elderly [9]. They often receive special attention from those who are involved with feeding programs for this group. However, evidence is lacking that psychological and sociological considerations are more important for the elderly than for other age groups.

Table 12–2
Frequency of Reported Eating Occasions in a Day

Sex and Age (Years)	*Number of Subjects Surveyed*	*Number of Eating Occasions per Day (%)*[a] 2	3	4	5	*Percentage of Subjects Eating Breakfast*
Males						
23-34	770	13	36	25	14	75
65-74	295	5	45	32	11	95
75+	127	8	58	24	4	98
Females						
23-34	949	10	39	25	14	76
65-74	377	6	54	28	9	96
75+	197	6	58	22	11	98

Source: Nationwide Food Consumption Survey, Spring 1977 [3]. Based on 24-hour recalls.
[a]Percentage of subjects who reported this frequency of eating occasions in a day. Does not add up to 100% due to the response categories not shown.

Eating Patterns

There are several studies suggesting that the elderly have more regular eating habits than do younger adults. Slesinger and colleagues [10], in studying a cross-section of the population of Milwaukee County, Wisconsin, observed that people over the age of 55 skipped fewer meals and that those over the age of 65 did less snacking than did younger people. In the recent U.S.D.A. Nationwide Food Consumption Survey [3], similar observations were made. Table 12-2 presents a comparison of meal eating between young and old adults in the U.S.D.A. survey. It is noteworthy that a major difference is the fact that most of the elderly eat breakfast. Less snacking by the elderly was also observed in this survey.

Food Patterns

In many comparisons, healthy elderly people, though they have reduced food intake, appear to select foods of somewhat higher nutritional quality than do younger adults. Slesinger and colleagues [10] reported that milk and meat intake decreased with age, particularly for women. Conversely, intake of fruits and vegetables and of breads and cereals increased.

In the Nationwide Food Consumption survey, more elderly people reported consumption of fruits, breads and cereals, vegetables, and milk (Table 12-3). Though the same numbers consumed meat, the elderly con-

Table 12–3
Use of Various Food Groups by Adults in a Day

Sex and Age (Years)	*Number of Subjects Surveyed*	*Milk (%)*[a]	*Breads (%)*[b]	*Cereals (%)*[c]	*Fruits (%)*	*Salads and Vegetables (%)*[d]
Males						
23-34	770	54	80	28	46	38
65-74	295	70	87	56	62	47
75 +	127	66	85	56	63	51
Females						
23-34	949	54	73	29	48	42
65-74	377	67	85	51	69	47
75 +	197	71	87	55	65	43

Source: Nationwide Food Consumption Survey, Spring 1977 [3]. Based on 24-hour recalls.
[a]Fluid milk.
[b]Breads, rolls, and biscuits.
[c]Cereals and pastas (includes ready-to-eat cereals).
[d]Includes tomatoes and dark green and deep yellow vegetables.

Table 12–4
Consumption of Meat by Adults

Sex and Age (Years)	*Number of Subjects Surveyed*	*Percentage Consuming Meat*[a]	*Amount Consumed (g)*[b]
Males			
23-34	770	94	305
65-74	295	95	244
75 +	127	95	207
Females			
23-34	949	90	203
65-74	377	92	172
75 +	197	91	148

Source: Nationwide Food Consumption Survey, Spring 1977 [3]. Based on 24-hour recalls.
[a]Percentage of subjects reporting consumption of meat, poultry, or fish in a day.
[b]Average intake in a day per person using meat.

sumed smaller amounts of meat (Table 12-4). The nutrient intake per 1,000 calories was generally increased in the elderly (Table 12-5). The intake of vitamins A and C directly correlates with the intake of fruits and vegetables. In this survey the elderly had better intakes of these vitamins than did young

Table 12–5
Nutrients per 1,000 Kilocalories for U.S. Adults

Sex and Age (Years)	*Number of Subjects Surveyed*	*Energy in Total Diet (kcal)*[a]	*Ca (mg)*	*Fe (mg)*	*Mg (mg)*	*Vitamin B_6 (mg)*	*Vitamin A (IU)*	*Vitamin C (mg)*
Males								
23-34	770	2,449	347	7	129	0.7	2,258	41
65-74	295	1,970	376	8	152	0.8	3,625	54
75+	127	1,808	387	8	154	0.9	3,833	54
Females								
23-34	949	1,616	384	7	143	0.8	2,920	54
65-74	377	1,444	406	8	164	0.9	4,659	70
75+	197	1,367	443	8	160	0.9	4,683	68

Source: Nationwide Food Consumption Survey, Spring 1977 [3]. Based on 24-hour recalls.
[a]Average intake for the group.

adults (see Table 12-1), correlating with their greater use of fruits and vegetables. This is in contrast to findings of low vitamin A intake in some elderly groups, particularly Spanish-American groups. Evidence obtained in these special groups has frequently been overgeneralized, and it has commonly been said that intake of vitamins A and C is low in the elderly. The evidence does not support this conclusion.

A comparison of total nutrient intake of the elderly to that of young adults suggests that the elderly on the average meet recommended intakes as well or better than young adults. For all adults, the average intakes of calcium, vitamin B_6, and magnesium are low compared to recommended intakes. Iron intakes (about 10-11 mg) are low for younger women, but the same intake is believed to be adequate for postmenopausal women. The evidence supports the view that food choices and nutrient intake are remarkably similar across different age groups [11].

Summary and Recommendations

1. The elderly differ from young adults in that they are more apt to eat breakfast and less apt to snack. Consideration of this regularity in eating is helpful when feeding or counseling the elderly.

2. Though calorie consumption is somewhat decreased, consumption of other nutrients is similar across all age groups. A higher intake of calcium, vitamin B_6, magnesium, and iron can be recommended for all adults.

3. Individual variability within any age group, but especially among the elderly, must be considered in effective counseling of individuals.

Counseling should be guided as little as possible by generalized assumptions.

4. Careful attention should be given to recommendations concerning nutrient supplementation for the elderly. Low food intakes coupled with increased numbers of individuals who have gastrointestinal problems or infections or other diseases lead to the observation that some elderly people could benefit from appropriate supplementation. The elderly should be counseled on an individual basis about the use of supplements.

References

1. *Ten-State Nutrition Survey, 1968*–1970: Highlights. D.H.E.W. Pub. no. (HSM) 72-8134, 1972.

2. *Dietary Intake Findings, United States, 1971–1974.* Data from the National Health Survey. D.H.E.W. Pub. no. (HRA) 77-1647, 1977.

3. Food and nutrient intakes of individuals in 1 day in the United States, Spring, 1977. U.S.D.A. Nationwide Food Consumption Survey, 1977–1978. Prelim. Rep. no. 2, 1980.

4. *Dietary Intake Findings, United States, 1977–1980.* Data from the National Health Survey, D.H.E.W. National Center for Health Statistics, preliminary data, 1982.

5. Exton-Smith, A.M. Eating habits of the elderly. In Turner, M. (Ed.), *Nutrition and Lifestyles.* London: Applied Science Publishers, 1980. P. 179.

6. Munro, H.N. Major gaps in nutrient allowances. The status of the elderly. *J. Am. Diet. Assoc.* 76:137–141, 1980.

7. Read, M.H., Graney, A.S. Food supplement usage by the elderly. *J. Am. Diet. Assoc.* 80:250–253, 1982.

8. Grandjean, A.C., Korth, L.L., Kara, G.C., et al. Nutrition status of elderly participants in a congregate meals program. *J. Am. Diet. Assoc.* 78:324–329, 1981.

9. Krondl, M., Lau, D., Yurkew, M.A., Coleman, P.H. Food use and perceived food meanings of the elderly. *J. Am. Diet. Assoc.* 80:523–529, 1982.

10. Slesinger, D.P., McDivitt, M., O'Donnell, F.M. Food patterns in an urban population: Age and sociodemographic correlates. *J. Gerontol.* 35:432–441, 1980.

11. Windham, C.T., Wyse, B.W., Hurst, R.L., Hansen, R.G. Consistency of nutrient consumption patterns in the United States. *J. Am. Diet. Assoc.* 78:587–595, 1981.

13 Nutritional Factors in Chronic Disease

Stephen P. Fortmann, M.D.

It is now widely appreciated that chronic diseases have assumed the greatest importance in the health of developed countries such as the United States. With improvement in the public health and welfare during the first three-quarters of this century, the number of people dying of acute, infectious diseases has steadily fallen, while the number dying of chronic diseases has steadily increased. This phenomenon is reflected in the contrast between life expectancy at birth, which has increased markedly during the 1900s, and life expectancy at age 45, which changed very little prior to the 1970s. The major causes of death in the United States are now cardiovascular diseases, cancer, and alcoholism. In 1978, for example, 665,000 persons aged 55-84 died of cardiovascular diseases, while 301,000 died from cancer. Arthritis, hypertension, and diabetes are also major chronic diseases in the middle-aged and elderly population in the United States. While these diseases contribute to mortality figures only indirectly, they are a major source of disability in this age group.

To some degree, nutritional factors are important in all of these conditions. Dietary fat, cholesterol, fiber, and calories contribute to cardiovascular diseases and cancer. Obesity and other nutritional factors contribute to hypertension and diabetes. Alcoholism has profound nutritional consequences. Even arthritis may be aggravated by obesity. Since the relationship of cancer to diet has already been reviewed in this symposium, and since hypertension and diabetes cause disability and death primarily through contributing to cardiovascular diseases, I will discuss the link between nutrition and heart disease.

I will begin by briefly reviewing the major risk factors for cardiovascular disease and summarizing the relationship of nutrition to some of them. I will then group nutritional factors into high, moderate, low, and negative atherogenic potential and discuss each in turn. I will close by summarizing the content of the prudent diet and the role of health professionals in disseminating nutritional information.

Cardiovascular Disease Risk Factors

The six major risk factors for cardiovascular disease are summarized in Table 13-1. Cigarette smoking, plasma low-density lipoprotein (LDL) (or total)

Table 13–1
Major Cardiovascular Disease Risk Factors

Factor	*Association*
Cigarette smoking	Positive
Plasma LDL cholesterol	Positive
Plasma HDL cholesterol	Negative
Arterial blood pressure	Positive
Obesity	Positive
Physical activity	Negative

LDL = low-density lipoprotein; HDL = high-density lipoprotein.

cholesterol, arterial blood pressure, and obesity are positively associated with the incidence of cardiovascular disease; that is, the higher the level of these factors, the greater is the risk of subsequent heart disease. In contrast, plasma HDL cholesterol and physical activity are negatively associated with heart and vascular diseases; people with high levels of high-density lipoprotein (HDL) levels or those who exercise regularly develop less disease.

The role of lipoprotein cholesterol is central to the development of cardiovascular disease. Cholesterol, triglyceride, and other lipids are insoluble in water and must be transported in the blood attached to protein molecules. There are four of these lipoprotein particles: chylomicrons, very-low-density lipoprotein (VLDL), low-density lipoprotein, and high-density lipoprotein. Chylomicrons are manufactured in the intestine and disappear between meals, while VLDL particles are manufactured in the liver (both of these particles transport triglyceride). Low-density lipoprotein is the major cholesterol-transporting particle, while the role of the small HDL is incompletely understood. Most epidemiologic studies have measured total cholesterol rather than lipoprotein cholesterol. The association between total cholesterol and coronary heart disease (CHD) is strongly positive. The majority of total cholesterol is found in the LDL particle, and it is this particle that crosses the arterial wall and forms atherosclerotic plaques. However, at least in societies where blood levels of LDL are excessive, the HDL particle is apparently protective and may be involved in removing cholesterol from arterial walls. Since LDL and HDL have opposite effects on atherogenesis, I will talk about them separately in this discussion.

Figure 13-1 shows the relationship of nutrition to cardiovascular disease (CVD) risk factors. Central to this web of causation is high LDL cholesterol, since an excess of this lipoprotein is necessary for atherogenesis. Unfortunately, an average U.S. cholesterol level (210 mg/dl) provides an ample amount of LDL for extensive atheroma formation. Obesity, excessive dietary fat and cholesterol, and low dietary fiber all contribute to elevated levels of LDL cholesterol. Obesity is also indirectly related to cardiovascular disease

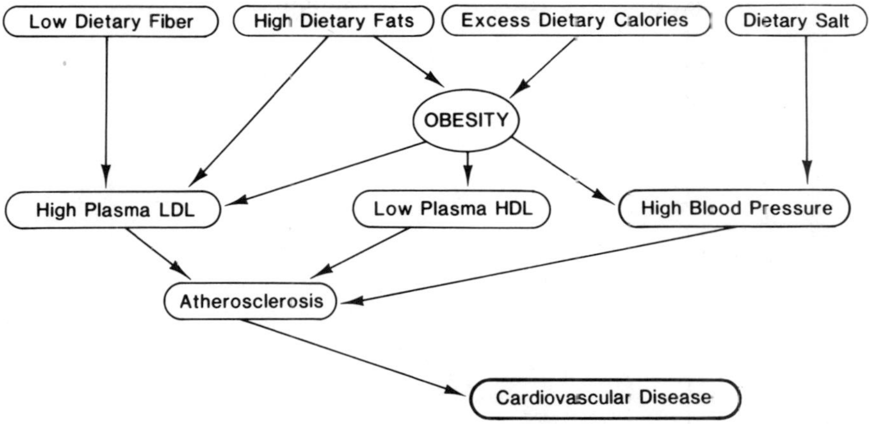

Figure 13-1. Theoretical web of causation connecting various nutritional factors to atherogenesis and cardiovascular disease. LDL = low-density lipoprotein; HDL = high-density lipoprotein.

through promoting low levels of HDL and high levels of blood pressure. Obesity may also contribute directly to cardiovascular disease, independent of its effects on the other three factors, but this hypothesis remains unsettled. However, as Figure 13-1 illustrates, the importance of obesity is undeniable. Finally, excessive dietary salt is shown to contribute to elevations in blood pressure. I will review all these factors in the following discussion.

The relationship between any of these factors and the risk of cardiovascular disease is shown in Figure 13-2. This example is for systolic blood pressure and risk of coronary heart disease in 12 years, but a similar figure could be shown for LDL cholesterol, cigarette smoking, or obesity. Note that the relationship is smooth and continuous, and that there is no point below which risk no longer falls. For this reason, optimal levels of many of these risk factors are below the average levels in this country. This means that the prevention of cardiovascular diseases is a problem for most people in society, not merely for a small, high-risk group [1].

Nutritional Factors of High Atherogenic Potential

Saturated fat and cholesterol intake, which may be examined together, and obesity are the two factors of high atherogenic potential. Dietary saturated fat and cholesterol contribute to the development of cardiovascular diseases by causing an increase in LDL cholesterol. Recalling Figure 13-1, it is possible to investigate the link between dietary fat and CVD by examining the relationship of diet to LDL cholesterol, LDL cholesterol to CVD, or diet to

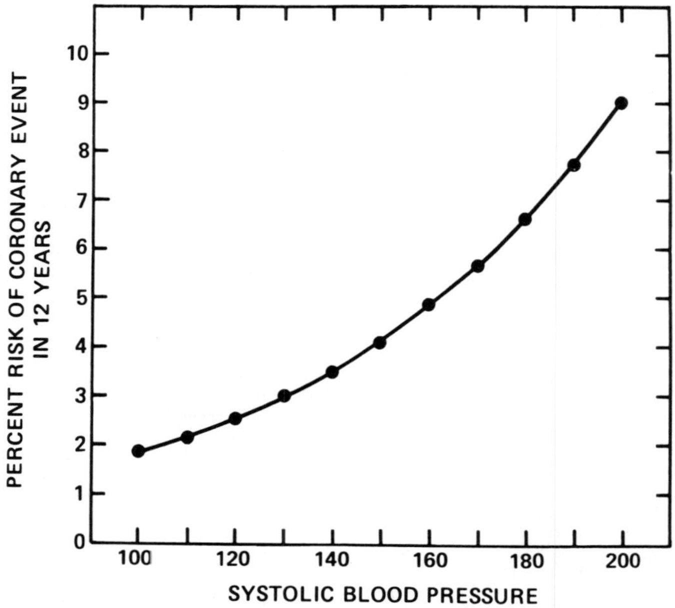

Figure 13-2. Relationship of systolic blood pressure (varying from 100 to 200 mm Hg) to the risk of a coronary event during a 12-year period for a 40-year-old male with serum cholesterol 220 mg/dl, relative weight 1.0.

CVD. All three links in this chain have been investigated in studies using one of four major methods: observational epidemiology, clinical research, animal models, or experimental epidemiology.

Observational epidemiology studies have examined the three links both by comparing different cultures and by comparing different people within one culture. The cross-cultural studies show that those areas of the world with high intakes of saturated fat and cholesterol also have high plasma cholesterol levels and CHD rates [2,3]. In Japan, for example, the diet is quite low in fat, the average total cholesterol is about 160 mg/dl, and heart disease rates are quite low. Eastern Finland, where the average cholesterol level is 270 mg/dl, has the highest coronary disease rates in the world. These cross-cultural studies clearly establish CVD to be environmentally determined; that diet is one environmental factor is strongly suggested. The advantage of cross-cultural studies is that they can examine a broad range of dietary intakes. A disadvantage is that many other environmental factors also differ among cultures, which may confound the diet-cholesterol-CHD analysis. Standardization of methods may also be difficult.

Some of these problems are lessened by single-culture epidemiologic studies. Many of these studies have shown a strong, consistent, positive association between plasma cholesterol and CHD incidence [4-6]. Such studies have shown less consistent relationships between diet and plasma cholesterol or between diet and heart disease than have cross-cultural studies. However, such relationships are much harder to demonstrate within a single culture, where the range of dietary intake is much smaller, given the difficulty of precisely characterizing diet [7]. The possibility of not detecting a true relationship becomes quite large; several epidemiologic studies have failed to show a relationship between dietary fat and either cholesterol or CHD [8]. However, one large study did show a relationship and also analyzed the role of dietary change in reducing the power of such studies [9,10]. Finally, autopsy studies [11] and angiographic studies [12] have demonstrated a clear association between plasma cholesterol and atheroma.

Some of these problems are surmounted by the second major line of evidence, clinical research. These studies examine the relationship between diet and plasma cholesterol in controlled settings, such as a metabolic ward. More than 30 years of these studies indicate a strong and consistent relationship between dietary saturated fat and plasma cholesterol. Though less important than saturated fat, dietary cholesterol is also a determinant of plasma cholesterol. These studies have resulted in mathematical formulas for predicting the changes in plasma cholesterol that will result from changes in dietary saturated fat or cholesterol [13].

The third major line of evidence is animal studies. In several animal models, it is possible to manipulate LDL cholesterol by increasing dietary saturated fat and cholesterol. These animals develop arterial plaques that are very similar to atherosclerosis in humans [14].

Epidemiologic experiments form the final line of evidence. In these studies, either the diet or plasma cholesterol is manipulated in a large number of free-living individuals who are then examined for the effects on either plasma cholesterol or coronary heart disease. Such studies have clearly shown that reductions in dietary saturated fat and cholesterol result in reductions in plasma cholesterol in such free-living individuals just as in the clinical research cited above [15,16]. There have also been several studies of dietary manipulations that have examined the development of CHD as the outcome. All of these studies had design problems, including short duration and small numbers of subjects, and all were inconclusive [16,17]. However, none were inconsistent with the hypothesis that diet is a causal factor in the development of CHD. A recent report of one European trial [18], where diet change and smoking cessation were combined, further strengthens the causal hypothesis.

The controversies that have surrounded diet and CHD during the past several years have focused on the incomplete evidence relating diet to CHD and on the issue of whether or not dietary cholesterol is an important factor in determining plasma cholesterol. These controversies result from isolating a small part of the broad spectrum of evidence discussed here. It is a difficult research proposition to demonstrate an association between diet and the development of CHD in single-culture studies. Some observers have overemphasized this area of research, forgetting that the absence of proof is not proof of absence. These studies are quite consistent with what is known about diet, plasma cholesterol, and heart disease. There is no doubt that diet is an important determinant of plasma cholesterol in a majority of people and that plasma cholesterol is a strong and consistent risk factor for CHD. It is highly likely that diet-induced reductions in plasma cholesterol do lower the risk of CHD.

The dietary cholesterol–plasma cholesterol controversy has centered on the egg. The egg is one of the few sources of dietary cholesterol that is not also high in saturated fat. Few serious observers have suggested that dietary saturated fat is unrelated to plasma cholesterol, but there have been studies showing that the addition of two or three eggs per day to the usual U.S. diet results in little change in plasma cholesterol in free-living individuals. This apparent contradiction with the clinical research on dietary and plasma cholesterol could be explained if the individuals changed other factors in their diet, either consciously or unconsciously, when they increased their egg intake. This possibility was examined in a recent study [19] in which the addition of eggs or egg substitute was performed in a double-blind fashion. In this study, increased dietary cholesterol was consistently associated with increased plasma cholesterol.

A prospective clinical trial of the diet–heart disease theory is not feasible, primarily because it would require too many years, subjects, and dollars. We must draw conclusions from *all* available evidence without retreating behind what is not known. The available evidence on this topic is highly suggestive that dietary modification to reduce plasma cholesterol would reduce the incidence of CVD.

Obesity may or may not be an independent, *direct* risk factor for the development of cardiovascular disease, but it is an important indirect risk factor through its effect on LDL cholesterol, blood pressure, and HDL cholesterol. Obesity is often considered a nutritional disease, since it is presumed to result from high caloric intake. While caloric excess is a factor in causing some obesity, in many people a more important factor is physical inactivity. Physicians are accustomed to seeing massively overweight individuals, some of whom do eat excessively (often in binges). However, the average American becomes overweight gradually with age and never seeks medical attention, since we consider this a rather normal process. Indeed, people who are at ideal weight, especially men, appear rather thin to our obesity-accustomed eyes. The average American is about 18 percent overweight, and nearly four out of five individuals exceed their ideal weight by at least 10 percent. However, per capita calorie intake has declined in this country since 1900, and it is likely that the parallel decline in physical activity is actually responsible for a greater part of the obesity in our society.

Nevertheless, foods that are concentrated in calorie content and relatively devoid of other nutritional value do contribute to obesity. These foods are ones that are high in fat and in sugar, both of which can pack a lot of calories in a mouthful. Thus, decreases in dietary fat and in refined sugar would likely contribute to a decrease in obesity and, in turn, to a lower risk of cardiovascular disease.

Nutritional Factors of Moderate Atherogenic Potential

I have included only one factor as being of moderate atherogenic potential, dietary sodium. The major dietary source of sodium is common salt, and the association with CVD is through elevations of blood pressure. There is again a broad range of evidence that links dietary sodium to blood pressure. Observational epidemiologic studies, both cross-cultural [20] and single-culture [21], have shown relationships between dietary sodium and blood pressure. Once again, determination of dietary sodium is difficult [22], and some single-culture studies have failed to show a consistent relationship. However, the studies that do show significant associations between salt intake and blood pressure level tend to be the ones with more careful measurement of dietary sodium. Some of the best work in this area has been performed by Liu and associates, who measured overnight urinary sodium on several occasions and found a significant association with blood pressure even in normotensive children [23].

There have also been numerous clinical studies which show that manipulations of dietary sodium will affect blood pressure in both hypertensive and normotensive individuals. It is well established that extremely low sodium diets (less than 10 mEq per day) will lower blood pressure in most individuals. There have also been several studies with moderate restrictions in sodium intake, down to about 70 mEq per day, with subsequent fall in blood pressure [24,25]. Some individuals are more sensitive to sodium change than others.

Finally, animal studies also suggest a relationship between dietary salt and arterial pressure. Several strains of rats have been bred to be sensitive to sodium in the diet, developing sustained hypertension even after brief exposure to high sodium intake during weaning. This susceptibility to dietary sodium seems to reside in the kidneys of these animals, and the presumed mechanism is an inability to handle excessive dietary salt without increasing blood pressure. These studies are consistent with an interaction between dietary sodium and heredity that would explain the pattern of sodium response in humans.

Nutritional Factors of Low Atherogenic Potential

Dietary caffeine and alcohol have some potential for increasing the likelihood of cardiovascular disease. Caffeine is a potent releaser of catecholamines, and the equivalent of two cups of coffee can raise systolic pressure 10–15 mm Hg and diastolic pressure 5–10 mm Hg [26]. However, the effects of long-duration exposure to caffeine are less well understood; it is possible that the cardiovascular system adapts to regular caffeine use. It has not been shown that coffee or other sources of methylxanthines are positively associated with cardiovascular disease.

The evidence on alcohol is even more controversial. Several studies have shown that alcoholics or individuals consuming more than about four drinks per day have higher blood pressure than people consuming less alcohol [27]. However, other studies have shown lower rates of coronary heart disease in individuals who are drinking about two drinks per day compared to individuals who never drink alcohol [28]. It has also been demonstrated that this modest level of alcohol use is associated with higher levels of HDL cholesterol [29].

Nutritional Factors of Negative Atherogenic Potential

There is also some good news when one is examining diet and heart disease. There are two nutrients that we should be eating more of, complex carbohydrates (or starch) and fiber. The link between complex carbohydrates and CHD is relatively weak but may be important since reductions in dietary fat must result in increases in dietary starch [8]. Complex carbohydrates, unlike simple sugars, decrease VLDL and insulin levels. This is particularly important in diabetics, who may actually experience a decreased insulin need and decreased blood sugar in response to certain complex carbohydrates in the diet [30,31]. Although VLDL is not thought to be atherogenic, it is possible that transient postprandial lipoprotein particles do result from high-sugar meals, and some researchers have postulated that these factors could be highly atherogenic [32].

Dietary fiber has achieved great notoriety during the past several years. This has resulted from several factors, including a possible relationship between low-fiber diets and colonic diverticulosis and cancer. Recent research on dietary fiber has shown that it lowers plasma LDL cholesterol and lowers insulin levels [33,34]. Most likely, fibers such as guar and pectin form gels in the intestine which trap cholesterol (i.e., bile acids) and sweep it out of the body. This is exactly the mechanism of the major drugs available for treating hypercholesterolemia, such as cholestyramine. In addition, these gels may isolate the bile acids from contact with bacteria in the colon. Certain bile acids may be converted to carcinogenic compounds by bacterial actions.

The Prudent Diet

This brief summary of some 30 years of research into the role of macronutrients in the cause of cardiovascular disease is necessarily superficial and is organized to emphasize the topic of atherogenesis. It is possible, however, to distill these several lines of research into a recommended "prudent diet." "Prudent" is used to acknowledge that the suggestions are reasonable extensions of what is known but that comprehensive clinical trials of the efficacy of this diet are absent. Table 13-2 shows the seven components of the prudent diet. We should all be eating a wide variety of foods to ensure adequate intake of essential micronutrients. We should work to maintain ideal weight; avoid too much fat, saturated fat, and cholesterol in the diet; and eat foods with adequate starch and fiber. We should look to decreasing sugar and sodium and to drinking alcohol only in moderation.

One might ask whether these dietary recommendations are appropriate for all members of society or only for high-risk individuals. This diet may be recommended to everyone. The relationship between nutritional risk factors and coronary heart disease is smooth and continuous. The CVD problem in the United States is not limited to a few high-risk individuals but rather is one of mass hyperlipidemia [35]; the average American dies of cardiovascular disease or cancer, in many cases prematurely. Americans would benefit from a diet that is lower in fat, cholesterol, and sugar and higher in carbohydrates and fiber.

Table 13-2
Components of a Prudent Diet

Eat a variety of foods
Maintain ideal weight
Decrease fat, saturated fat, and cholesterol intake
Increase starch and fiber intake
Reduce refined sugar intake
Reduce sodium intake
Drink alcohol in moderation

Nor is this diet particularly new. It is much closer to the diet eaten by preindustrial man and possibly resembles the one on which we evolved for a long period of time. It resembles diets common in Asia and the Mediterranean even today. These facts support the safety of the recommendations.

In addition, our diet is continually manipulated by the food industry for purposes of profit. Various economic forces also change dietary habits. So to say nothing about diet is, in fact, to advocate these changes—changes that have often included increased amounts of fat, sugar, and salt. Why should physicians and nutritional scientists refrain from telling the public what is known about nutrition and chronic disease? To leave such a void is to invite it to be filled by much less responsible forces.

Role of Health Professionals

Does this information have any practical importance for most practicing health professionals? Is not advice on diet the purview of public health professionals? Can physicians have any impact on their patients' diet? First, it is important to realize that dietary change will occur gradually in society and in one's patients. It is all too easy in clinical practice to become discouraged with the issues of weight control, smoking cessation, and dietary change. However, we are at the disadvantage of trying to achieve rapid change in people who are often clinically ill or who represent the extreme end of the problem. The steady flow of information to the general public, emanating from doctors directly and the health professions in general, can be important. The example of cigarette smoking is pertinent. Although we have all been frustrated at trying to get a patient who desperately needs to quit smoking to do so, the steady flow of information over the last 20 years about the dangers of smoking has had an effect. Every measure of cigarette consumption has shown a steady decline in the last decade and a half, including the proportion of the population smoking and per capita cigarette use. While we often are confronted with our impotence, we should remember that physicians and other health professionals are, in fact, among the most potent change agents for many people.

Thus, in your practice you can begin by not ignoring the problem. Be certain to weigh patients and warn those who are overweight or who are steadily gaining. Of course, measure blood pressure and assess smoking cessation and diet. Your advice can be brief and augmented by numerous written materials that are available from the federal government and the American Heart Association. Things will not change overnight, and we will continue to collect research data about nutrition and chronic disease, but the medical profession can be a leader in achieving improved health through improved nutrition.

Summary

The major risk factors for cardiovascular disease have been reviewed, and the relationship of nutrition to some of these has been summarized. Nutritional factors can be grouped according to their atherogenic potential.

Dietary intake of saturated fat and cholesterol is associated with high atherogenic potential by contributing to the development of cardiovascular diseases through an increase in low-density-lipoprotein cholesterol. Obesity may not be an independent, *direct* risk factor for cardiovascular disease, but it is important indirectly through its effect on LDL cholesterol, blood pressure, and HDL cholesterol. Although calorie intake has declined in the United States, a parallel decline in physical activity may be responsible for much of the obesity in our society.

Dietary sodium can be regarded as a factor of moderate atherogenic potential. It is associated with cardiovascular disease through its elevation of blood pressure; both hypertensive and normotensive individuals are affected.

Low atherogenic potential can be assigned to caffeine and alcohol. The former is a potent stimulator of catecholamine secretion in the acute situation; however, the effects (or their lack) of long-term exposure to caffeine are less well understood. The evidence of the relationship between alcohol and blood pressure is controversial, but it suggests that less alcohol intake is associated with lower blood pressure.

Intake of both complex carbohydrates and fiber tends to reduce atherogenic potential. This may be of particular value for the diabetic patient.

A "prudent" diet has been suggested that ensures adequate intake of micronutrients, reduces intake of foods that have atherogenic potential, and increases intake of those foods that reduce atherogenic potential. In addition, the individual should strive to maintain ideal weight by regulating calorie intake and pursuing regular exercise.

The health professional must recognize that the dietary habits of the population change slowly. Nevertheless, the health professional can assume leadership in achieving improved health through improved nutrition: by monitoring patients' body weight, blood pressure, and diet; by providing to patients sound dietary advice backed by publications from the federal government and the American Heart Association; and by continuing to supply a steady flow of information on diet and health to the general public and to public policy makers.

References

1. Stamler, J. Lifestyles, major risk factors, proof, and public policy. *Circulation* 58:3–19, 1978.

2. Keys, A. *Seven Countries: A Multivariate Analysis of Death and Coronary Heart Disease*. Cambridge, Mass.: Harvard University Press, 1980.

3. Robertson, T.L., Kato, H., Gordon, T., et al. Epidemiological studies of CHD and stroke in Japanese men living in Japan, Hawaii and California. *Am. J. Cardiol.* 39:244–249, 1977.

4. Dawber, T.R. *The Framingham Study: The Epidemiology of Atherosclerotic Disease*. Cambridge, Mass.: Harvard University Press, 1980.

5. Pooling Project Research Group. Relationship of blood pressure, serum cholesterol, smoking habit, relative weight and ECG abnormalities to incidence of major coronary events: Final report of the Pooling Project. *J. Chronic Dis.* 31:201-306, 1978.

6. Rosenman, R.H., Brand, R.J., Sholtz, R.I., Friedman, M. Multivariate prediction of coronary heart disease during 8.5 year follow-up in the Western Collaborative Group Study. *Am. J. Cardiol.* 37:903–910, 1976.

7. Jacobs, R.R., Anderson, J.T., Blackburn, H. Diet and serum cholesterol: Do zero correlations negate the relationship? *Am. J. Epidemiol.* 110:77–87, 1979.

8. Gordon, T., Kagan, A., Garcia-Palmieri, M., et al. Diet and its relation to coronary heart disease and death in three populations. *Circulation* 63:500–515, 1981.

9. Shekelle, R.B., Shryock, A.M., Paul, O., et al. Diet, serum cholesterol, and death from coronary heart disease. *N. Engl. J. Med.* 304:65–70, 1981.

10. Shekelle, R.B., Stamler, J., Paul, O., et al. Dietary lipids and serum cholesterol level: Change in diet confounds the cross-sectional association. *Am. J. Epidemiol.* 115:506–514, 1982.

11. Rhoads, G.G., Blackwelder, W.C., Stemmermann, G.N., et al. Coronary risk factors and autopsy findings in Japanese-American men. *Lab. Invest.* 38:304–311, 1978.

12. Gotto, A.M., Gorry, G.A., Thompson, J.R., et al. Relationship between plasma lipid concentrations and coronary heart disease in 496 patients. *Circulation* 56:875–883, 1977.

13. Keys, A., Anderson, J.T., Grande, F. Serum cholesterol response to changes in the diet. *Metabolism* 14:747–758, 759–765, 1965.

14. Armstrong, M.C., Warner, E.D., Connor, W.E. Regression of coronary atheromatosis in rhesus monkeys. *Circ. Res.* 27:59–67, 1970.

15. Page, I.H., Brown, H.B. Some observations on the National Diet-Heart Study. *Circulation* 37:313–315, 1968.

16. Dayton, S., Pearce, M.C., Hashimoto, S., et al. A controlled clinical trial of a diet high in unsaturated fat. *Circulation* 39/40 (Suppl. 2):1–63, 1969.

17. Davis, C.E., Havlik, R.J. Clinical trials in lipid lowering and coronary artery disease prevention. In Rifkind, B.M., Levy, R.I. (Eds.), *Hyperlipidemia: Diagnosis and Therapy*. New York: Grune and Stratton, 1977. Pp. 79–92.

18. Hjermann, I., Holme, L., Byre, K.V., Leren, P. Effect of diet and smoking intervention on the incidence of coronary heart disease. *Lancet* 2:1303–1310, 1981.

19. Roberts, S.L., McMurray, M.P., Connor, W.E. Does egg feeding (i.e., dietary cholesterol) affect plasma cholesterol levels in humans? The results of a double-blind study. *Am. J. Clin. Nutr.* 34:2092–2099, 1981.

20. Prior, I.A.M., Evans, J.G. Harvey, H.P.B. et al. Sodium intake and blood pressure in two Polynesian populations. *N. Engl. J. Med.* 279:515–520, 1968.

21. Pietinen, P.I., Wong, O., Altschul, A.M. Electrolyte output, blood pressure, and family history of hypertension. *Am. J. Clin. Nutr.* 32:997–1005, 1979.

22. Liu, K., Cooper, R., McKeever, J., et al. Assessment of the association between habitual salt intake and high blood pressure: Methodological problems. *Am. J. Epidemiol.* 110:219–226, 1979.

23. Cooper, R., Soltero, I., Liu, K., et al. The association between urinary sodium excretion and blood pressure in children. *Circulation* 62:97–102, 1980.

24. Morgan, T., Gillies, A., Morgan, G., et al. Hypertension treated by salt restriction. *Lancet* 1:227–230, 1978.

25. MacGregor, G.A., Best, F.E., Cam, J.M., et al. Double-blind randomised cross-over trial of moderate sodium restriction in essential hypertension. *Lancet* 1:351-355, 1982.

26. Robertson, D., Frolich, J.C., Carr. K., et al. Effects of caffeine on plasma renin activity, catecholamines and blood pressure. *N. Engl. J. Med.* 298:181–186, 1978.

27. Klatsky, A.L., Friedman, G.D., Siegelaub, A.B., Gerard, M.J. Alcohol consumption and blood pressure. *N. Engl. J. Med.* 296:1194–1200, 1977.

28. Yano, K., Rhoads, G.G., Kagan, A. Coffee, alcohol and risk of coronary heart disease among Japanese men living in Hawaii. *N. Engl. J. Med.* 297:405–409, 1977.

29. Hulley, S.B., Gordon, S. Alcohol and high-density lipoprotein cholesterol. Causal inference from diverse study designs. *Circulation* 64 (Suppl. 3):57–62, 1981.

30. Coulston, A., Greenfield, M.S., Kraemer, F.B., et al. Effect of difference in source of dietary carbohydrate on plasma glucose and insulin responses to meals in patients with impaired carbohydrate tolerance. *Am. J. Clin. Nutr.* 34:2706–2710, 1981.

31. Crapo, P.A., Insel, J., Sperling, M., Kolterman, O.G. Comparison of serum glucose, insulin, and glucagon responses to different types of complex carbohydrate in noninsulin-dependent diabetic patients. *Am. J. Clin. Nutr.* 34:184–190, 1981.

32. Zilversmit, D.B. Atherogenesis: A postprandial phenomenon. *Circulation* 60:473–485, 1979.

33. Simpson, H.C.R., Lousley, S., Geekie, M., et al. A high carbohydrate leguminous fibre diet improves all aspects of diabetic control. *Lancet* 1:3–5, 1981.

34. Faser, F.E., Jacobs, D.R., Anderson, J.T., et al. The effect of various vegetable supplements on serum cholesterol. *Am. J. Clin. Nutr.* 34:1272–1277, 1981.

35. Blackburn, H.B. Diet and mass hyperlipidemia: A public health view. In Levy, R.I., Rifkind, B., Dennis, B., et al., (Eds.), *Nutrition, Lipids, and CHD.* New York: Raven Press, 1979. Pp. 309–347.

Discussion

Questions were addressed to the panel of speakers, which consisted of Dr. Gastineau, Dr. Swan, and Dr. Fortmann.

The discussion began with questions related to exercise and body weight reduction. It was pointed out that isometric exercises such as weight lifting against springs make very little demand on the cardiovascular system, and their usefulness is restricted to increasing muscle mass and strength. The type of exercise that makes demands on the cardiovascular system and also increases oxygen consumption will produce increased caloric expenditure. The distinction is based on the concept of aerobic demands. Thus, exercise that results in an increase in heart rate, in rate and depth of respiration, and in generating body heat is beneficial in controlling adiposity and possibly in the prevention of cardiovascular disease.

Obese patients on a body weight reduction program should be counseled about realistic expectations for weight loss. It is frequently forgotten that increased caloric expenditure due to exercise is the amount of calories used beyond those required for activities other than exercise. For example, a 150-pound individual walking at 2–4 miles per hour will burn about 50 calories more per mile than he would have burned sitting still. At this rate of caloric consumption, utilization of one pound of adipose tissue containing 3,500 calories will require 70 miles of walking. The patient should not expect too much from exercise, which may be disappointing. On the other hand, a combination of dietary management and mild daily exercise can lead an obese patient toward realistic rates of weight loss and better overall health.

Concerning the effectiveness of exercise, consistency is more beneficial than strenuousness. For most obese patients it is more advantageous to walk rather than to enter a jogging program, particularly since the caloric expenditure of walking is very close to that of jogging, on the basis of distance. Moreover, a consistent rate of weight loss is better from the viewpoint of emotional and physical health than the rhythm method of going up and down in body weight throughout one's life.

The other beneficial aspect of exercise has to do with the prevention of coronary disease. There is some evidence that physical fitness at the cardiovascular training level is associated with a lower risk of coronary disease independent of its effects on other risk factors. This effect appears to be a result of increasing the efficiency of the cardiovascular system. To achieve the training level, aerobic-type exercise should be performed for about 20 minutes three to four times per week at about 70 percent of the approximate theoretical maximum heart rate. Of course, the type of exercise needed to achieve this level will differ among individuals.

This panel, as did the others, suggested that the average U.S. diet is adequate in its nutritional and caloric content. There are, however, certain specific, circumscribed conditions when supplementation may be considered. These conditions have been discussed by previous speakers. The real danger with nutrition supplements is that rather remarkable imbalances can easily be achieved. Furthermore, high consumption of certain nutrients interferes with the function and use of other nutrients. This presents a particular danger in the elderly, since the group is also more likely to receive a variety of medications. Potential food and drug interactions should be of real concern in this population.

It should also be noted that in a free-living, healthy population, nutrient needs do not increase greatly with age. However, both the frequency of chronic diseases and the intake of medication do increase in an older population. Therefore, this population will demonstrate altered nutritional needs. On the basis of several studies, it also appears that the elderly may be slightly less efficient in the use of nitrogen. On the other hand, older people at the same weight have less lean body mass and therefore are turning over less protein per day. These two effects tend to cancel each other out such that if one recommends about the same amount of protein intake, the older person receives a slightly greater amount per kilogram of lean body mass. Thus the recommended daily allowances remain the same throughout life, and the elderly meet their slightly greater protein need for maintaining their lean body mass.

Concerning circulating cholesterol, the audience raised questions about its origin, the role of dietary cholesterol, and the effect of exercise on plasma cholesterol. As Dr. Fortmann explained, about half of total cholesterol is formed by the body, both in the liver and in the periphery. Much of that synthesis is regulated by plasma low-density lipoproteins (LDLs); it is shut off when the LDL concentration exceeds 40–50 mg/dl. In addition, certain genetic factors appear to determine plasma cholesterol and plasma high-density lipoprotein (HDL) levels, which have been suggested to have important roles in the regulation of plasma cholesterol concentration and in the transport of cholesterol to steroid-hormone-synthesizing cells. Nevertheless, on the epidemiologic level it is dietary cholesterol and saturated fat that produce toxic LDL levels in plasma.

Conversely, certain types of cancer appear to be correlated with lowered (less than normal) plasma cholesterol. However, these observations were made in studies that were designed neither to address this question directly nor to examine the physiologic consequences of lowered cholesterol levels. This area is suggested, therefore, as a fruitful and important direction for further investigation.

The important role of fluid intake and fluid balance in health maintenance has been well documented. Particularly in the elderly population, fluid requirements are often met with coffee, tea, or alcoholic beverages. Therefore the question was posed as to the possible nutritional effects of these substances. In addressing this question, the panel agreed that whereas coffee and tea have a diuretic effect, their use does not usually result in a significant effect on nutrition. Alcohol, in modest quantities, evokes complicated physiologic responses which can greatly affect nutrition in many different ways. There is no recommended daily allowance for alcohol. In a nutritional sense, there is a possibility that modest quantities, 100–150 calories per day, may have some protective effect against atherosclerotic heart disease. However, this effect is farther removed from having a likely causal relationship than a number of other factors.

It must be understood that alcohol is a toxin acting on the gastrointestinal tract and on the liver; it produces ketosis and it is a hypoglycemic agent in the diabetic. Furthermore, alcohol is a nutritional diluent, with as little as 10–20 percent of daily calories ingested as alcohol causing reduction in the nutritional density (in caloric terms) of the diet. Based on clinical experience, there is a suggestion that about 55 percent of daily caloric intake represents the maximum physiologic ability of the body to metabolize alcohol. Thus, both its toxic effects and its dilution of nutritional density lead to a progressive increase of the hazards of malnutrition with continued ingestion of alcohol.

As a last topic for discussion in this session on nutrition in the elderly, the question was raised as to the relationship between diet and senile dementia and presenile dementia (Alzheimer's disease). When confronted with these possibilities, it is important to differentiate them from early signs of pernicious anemia, which is often totally reversible by standard parenteral vitamin B_{12} therapy. There is a suggestion that aluminum excess may be related to facilitation of Alzheimer's disease. Nevertheless, there is very little definitive evidence that a dietary etiology exists for Alzheimer's disease.

V Food: Responsibilities and Goals

14 Medical Care and Nutrition for School-Age Children: Role of Physicians and Intervention Programs

Meinhard Robinow, M.D.

The School Health Team and Its Responsibilities

In discussing the school health team I shall limit myself to some current health and nutrition problems and to the responsibilities of those involved with intervention: the school physician and his or her supporting team, that is, the school nurse, food service supervisors, health and sex educators, biology teachers, home economics instructors, and athletic coaches. I speak as a pediatrician. School health and nutrition are major concerns of the Academy of Pediatrics and two of its permanent committees, the Committee on School Health and the Committee on Nutrition. The recommendations of these committees are published in *Pediatrics*, the monthly journal of the Academy. They are periodically brought out in book form as *School Health: A Guide for Health Professionals* [1] and *Pediatric Nutrition Handbook* [2].

It is the responsibility of local government, that is, health departments and boards of education, to ensure that appropriate school health services are provided. The *School Health Guide* [1] recommends a written contract between the school health board and the school physician which clearly delineates responsibilities and accountabilities for screening, for health, nutrition, and sex education, for supervision of athletic activities, for first aid, and for methods of reporting to parents. I strongly endorse such specific contracts.

Health of School-Age Children

Morbidity and mortality are high in the neonatal period, decline rapidly during infancy, reach a low at ages 10–14 years [3], and begin to rise again in adolescence, largely due to an increase in violent deaths (accidents, homicides, and suicides).

The superb health of today's children is partly a result of improved nutrition but mainly due to the virtual elimination of the life-threatening communicable diseases by public health measures, especially mass immunization. It is a major responsibility of the school physician and the school nurse to make sure that immunization requirements are complied with.

Accidents are now the leading cause of death in the school-age child. Their prevention must become a major concern of all school education programs.

Advantage of Screening Procedures over Conventional Physical Examination

The standard preschool physical examination rarely yields much information of value. It is certainly not cost-effective. Most important, school-age health and nutrition problems (incomplete immunizations, visual and auditory deficits, scoliosis, short stature, underweight, anemia, and so on) are more efficiently and more economically identified by school nurses. Several recent studies in Sweden and the United States [4–6] have quite impressively documented this point. The physician's time can be freed for more important duties, such as evaluation of students for contact sports, supervision of athletic programs, and, most important, the design of health, nutrition, and sex education programs.

All schools should have some schedule for initial health screening and periodic reevaluation. Requirements for kindergarten entrance might be as listed in Table 14-1. Height, weight, hearing, vision, and hemoglobin should be rechecked at predetermined intervals. Criteria for diagnosing abnormalities must be formulated and methods devised for informing parents without causing undue alarm and for making appropriate referrals. Confidentiality must be preserved.

Table 14–1
Proposed Requirements for Kindergarten Entry

Proof of completed immunizations
A parental statement concerning illnesses or handicaps requiring special care or restriction of activities
Vision and hearing screens
Height and weight measurements
Hemoglobin (or hematocrit) and free erythrocyte protoporphyrin (FEP), and blood lead levels for those with elevated FEP

Growth and Maturation of School-Age Children

The major national health and nutrition surveys [7–9] have shown that height, weight, and skeletal and sexual maturation of most U.S. children are very close to the means of the elite—that is, socioeconomically advantaged groups. Heights, weight, and skinfolds of children from families below the poverty level (income less that $800 per capita) averaged significantly lower [9,10]. However, the differences were small. In the case of height at age 10, they corresponded to the secular difference between 1960 and 1970 [9].

The secular increase of stature seems to have come to a halt [11,12], and the age of menarche is no longer advancing [12]. Today short stature, underweight, or delayed maturation usually result from diseases of digestion or metabolism, such as cystic fibrosis, regional enteritis, or renal disease, rather than from extrinsic conditions such as malnutrition due to poverty or otherwise inappropriate diets.

Deficiencies of Specific Nutrients in School-Age Children

The Ten-State Nutrition Survey [13] identified iron deficiency as the only common deficiency disorder of the young. Almost all the anemias were mild (hemoglobin, 10–12 g/dl). Whether mild iron deficiency, even in the absence of anemia, impairs health or interferes with learning ability remains a controversial issue [14–17]. But even mild iron deficiency should not be ignored; it reduces the margin of safety and thus represents a health concern that warrants periodic screening, especially in poverty areas. Nearly all other deficiencies of trace minerals and vitamins have now been eliminated by the introduction of fortified milk, enriched flour, iodized salt, and fluoridated water. I shall not discuss zinc nutriture. Too little is known about the prevalence of zinc deficiency to state whether it is a significant school health problem in the United States.

Nutritional Status of the Pregnant Teenager

The pregnant teenager presents a special and very difficult problem of school-age health care. Diets that are borderline or even adequate for the average teenage girl are likely to be insufficient for the pregnant teenager and her fetus. Moreover, unplanned pregnancy is more common among poor teenage girls whose prepregnancy diets are likely to have been poor. The shorter the interval between menarche and pregnancy, the greater is the risk of maternal complications and of unfavorable fetal outcome [18–21]. The malnourished young mother is also at a greatly increased risk of toxemia of pregnancy [22]. According to Beal [23], nearly 20 percent of all live-born infants in the United States with weights under 2.5 kg are born to mothers under 15 years of age. Most of these low birth weights are due to prematurity, not to intrauterine growth retardation [24]. These infants are at risk for all the problems of prematurity, especially the greatly increased mortality [18,21]. This is a problem of inadequate prenatal care. Physical immaturity of the very young mother is *not* a significant obstetric problem.

The poor results of unplanned teenage pregnancy are largely a socioeconomic problem. Semmens [25] showed that married teenagers below age 15 who lived at a U.S. naval base had, with few exceptions, a very satisfactory pregnancy outcome.

Some intervention programs in Baltimore, in New York City, and in Rochester, New York, have been successful in improving the outcome of teenage pregnancy [19,26,27]. Signs of progress can also be seen on a national scale. The rate of teenage pregnancy has dropped as much as the national birth rate [28], and there has been a recent decline in the rate of births to unmarried teenagers [28]. But the problems of teenage pregnancy continue to pose a difficult challenge to the school health team.

Current Dietary Patterns in Relation to Future Health and Longevity

Most nutritionists agree that the average American diet contains too many calories, too much fat, especially animal-derived fat, too much refined carbohydrate, too much meat, too much salt, excessive caloric density, and too little fiber. These excesses contribute to obesity with its many complications [29–31], gallbladder disease, non-insulin-dependent diabetes, dental caries, ischemic heart disease, hypertension, stroke, gout, and, almost certainly, to cancer of the colon, breast, and prostate [32–35]. Problems of abundance may now be more serious in the United States than the much publicized concerns over scarcities. Preventing ischemic heart disease and cancer in the middle years seems to me more important than achieving maximum growth and earliest maturation. After all, we are not fattening children for the market, as Jonathan Swift suggested 250 years ago as a solution to poverty [36].

The rapid growth and maturation induced by abundant food may be a doubtful gift to mankind. It has long been known that food restriction in laboratory animals, in farm animals, and, by inference, in humans, not only delays maturation but also prolongs the life span and decreases the incidence of cancer, heart disease, and kidney disease [37,38]. The accumulated evidence, indirect as it was, led the U.S. [39], Canadian [40], and British governments in 1977 to recommend substantial changes in the national diets. The wisdom and practicability of the recommendations have been questioned by some [41,42], but the public has listened and has modified its diet [43]. The death rate from ischemic heart disease and stroke has declined, although other factors (e.g., antihypertensive therapy) have contributed to this improvement.

Unfortunately, the composition of many school lunches is influenced more by the availability of surplus dairy products from the Department of Agriculture than by the newer insights concerning desirable nutrition. The interests of the meat and dairy industries are, of course, opposed to major changes in the American diet. The dairy industry has long tried to persuade the public that humans cannot be healthy without drinking the milk of another animal species. This is an absurd proposition from the anthropologic point of view. Still, there may be some truth to the slogan "You never outgrow the need for milk": if, as many people believe, high consumption of meat, with its high phosphorus and low calcium content, contributes to osteoporosis in later life, then milk may be a desirable though "unnatural" food to counteract the unfavorable calcium-phosphorus ratio of prevailing diets. Whether milk is necessary and advisable for the school-age child remains controversial [44]. We should remember that osteoporosis is extremely rare in some populations that eat little meat and drink no milk.

Achieving Improved Dietary Patterns and Healthier Life-Styles by Appropriate Education

Changes to a healthier life-style will not be made without education. Mann [29] wrote, "Children cannot rely on innate senses to make dietary choices. They must *learn* to use food appropriately." A committee of the American Heart Association [45] stated: "Nutrition education from kindergarten to high school will and should occur in settings other than school, but there are convincing reasons for making school the focal point." I would like to stress "kindergarten to high school"—that is, the need for continuity of health education and for coordination of programs between biology, health education, and physical education. Competitive sports, by the very nature of competition, exclude a large part of school-age children from participation. I would like to see more emphasis on noncompetitive athletic activities for the young, such as jogging or aerobic dancing. I believe we are moving in that direction.

We should avoid preaching and moralizing. We need teachers in our schools, not missionaries. The moralistic drug education programs in the schools have not significantly altered drug-taking behavior [46]. Dahl [47], in 1972, expressed it nicely: "I am convinced that adding salt is bad, but I do not think it a sin." Conversely, one might say that following a prudent diet and life-style promises health and longevity but does not lay up treasures in heaven.

Dietary patterns and life-styles are changing for the better [43,48], though perhaps not yet sufficiently for best results, as a recent report from Israel suggests [49]. The greatest improvements have taken place among the educated and the socioeconomically advantaged. People from the upper social classes exercise more and smoke less, and women from these classes are slimmer and are breast-feeding their infants again [50–52]. It is likely that social prestige ("you can never be too rich or too thin") plays as important a part as education. It may be easier to appeal to prestige than to common sense, as the advertising industry has always known. One may wonder what might happen to the prevalence of breast-feeding in Britain if Princess Diana could be seen on television breast-feeding the new heir to the British throne.

Summary

The health of today's children is superb. Mass immunizations have led to virtual elimination of life-threatening communicable diseases. Screening examinations effectively identify those with nutritional problems. The prevailing nutrition of school-age children ensures near-optimal growth and maturation for most U.S. children. A group that remains at high risk for nutritional deficiency are teenagers with unplanned pregnancy.

The average American diet, which results in healthy children, may threaten adult health and longevity due to its atherogenic properties and the possibility of contribution to an increased incidence of nonplastic disease. Improved dietary patterns and healthier life-styles can be achieved through educational programs.

References

1. Committee on School Health, American Academy of Pediatrics. *School Health: A Guide for Health Professionals.* Evanston, Ill.: American Academy of Pediatrics, 1977.

2. Committee on Nutrition, Academy of Pediatrics. *Pediatric Nutrition Handbook.* Evanston, Ill.: American Academy of Pediatrics, 1979.

3. Vaughn, V.C. In Vaughn, V.C., McNay, R.J., Behrman, R.E. (Eds.), *Textbook of Pediatrics*, 11th ed. Philadelphia: W.B. Saunders, 1979. P. 3.

4. Grant, W.W., Farnow, R.G., Hebertson, L.M., Henderson, A.L. Health screening in school-age children. *Am. J. Dis. Child.* 125:520–522, 1973.

5. Köhler, L. Physical mass examinations in the school health service. *Acta Paediatr. Scand.* 66:304–310, 1977.

6. Welch, N.M., Saulsbury, F.T., Kesler, R.W. The value of preschool examination in screening for health problems. *J. Pediatr.* 100:232–234, 1982.

7. U.S. Department of Health, Education and Welfare. *Ten-State Nutrition Survey.* D.H.E.W. no. (HSM) 72:8132, 1972.

8. Hamill, P.V.V., Drizd, T.A., Johnson, C.L., et al. *NCHS Growth Curves for Children Birth–18 Years.* D.H.E.W. Publication no. (PHS) 78–1650.

9. Hamill, P.V.V., Johnston, P.E., Lemeshow, S., et al. Physical growth: National Center for Health Statistics percentiles. *Am. J. Clin. Nutr.* 32:607–629, 1979.

10. Garn, S.M., Clark, D.C. Nutrition, growth, development, and maturation: Findings from the Ten-State Nutrition Survey of 1968-1970. *Pediatrics* 56:306–319, 1975.

11. Bakwin, H., McLaughlin, S. Secular increase in height: Is the end in sight? *Lancet* 2:1195–1196, 1964.

12. Damon, A. Larger body size and earlier menarche: The end may be in sight. *Soc. Biol.* 21:8–11, 1974.

13. *Ten-State Nutrition Survey 1968–1970: Highlights.* D.H.E.W. Publication no. (HMS) 72:8134, 1972.

14. Pollitt, E., Leibel, R.L. Iron deficiency and behavior. *J. Pediatr.* 88:372–381, 1976.

15. Leibel, R.L. Behavioral and biochemical correlates of iron deficiency. *J. Am. Diet. Assoc.* 71:398–404, 1977.

16. Read, M.S. Malnutrition, hunger and behavior: I. Malnutrition and learning. *J. Am. Diet. Assoc.* 63:379–385, 1973.

17. Webb, T.E., Oski, F.A. Iron deficiency anemia and scholastic achievement in young adolescents. *J. Pediatr.* 82:827–830, 1973.

18. Grant, J.A., Heald, F.P. Complications of adolescent pregnancy. Survey of the literature on fetal outcome in adolescence. *Clin. Pediatr.* 11:567–570, 1972.

19. Heald, F.P., Jacobson, M.S. Nutritional need of the pregnant adolescent. *Pediatr. Ann.* 9:59–99, 1980.

20. Armstrong, R.J. *A Study of Infant Mortality from Linked Records by Birthweight, Period of Gestation, and Other Variables, United States.* Vital and Health Statistics Series 20, no. 12. D.H.E.W. Publication no. (HSM) 72–1055, 1972.

21. Niswander, K., Jackson, E.C. Physical characteristics of the gravida and their association with birth weight and perinatal death. *Am. J. Obstet. Gynecol.* 119:306–313, 1974.

22. Brewer, T.H. *Metabolic Toxemia of Late Pregnancy: A Disease of Malnutrition.* Springfield: Ill.: Charles C Thomas, 1966.

23. Beal, V.A. *Nutrition in the Life Span.* New York: John Wiley and Sons, 1980.

24. Merritt, T.A., Lawrence, R.A., Naye, R.L. The infants of adolescent mothers. *Pediatr. Ann.* 9:100–110, 1980.

25. Semmens, J.P. *Teen-age Pregnancy.* Springfield, Ill.: Charles C Thomas, 1968.

26. McAnarney, E.R., Roghman, K.J., Adams, B.N., et al. Obstetric, neonatal, and psychologic outcome of pregnant adolescents. *Pediatrics* 61:199–206, 1977.

27. Field, T., Widmayer, S., Stringer, S., et al. Teenage, lower class black mothers and their preterm infants: An intervention and developmental follow-up. *Child Dev.* 51:426–436, 1980.

28. Monthly Vital Statistics Report. *Final Natality Statistics, 1978.* D.H.H.S. Publication no. (PHS) 80–1120, vol. 29, no. 1, Suppl., April 28, 1980.

29. Mann, G.V. The influence of obesity on health. *N. Engl. J. Med.* 291:178–185, 226–232, 1974.

30. Kannell, W.B., Brand, N., Skinner, J.J., et al. Relation of adiposity to blood pressure and the development of hypertension: The Framingham study. *Ann. Intern. Med.* 67:48–59, 1967.

31. Heyden, S., Hames, C.G., Bartel, A., et al. Weight and weight history in relation to cardiovascular and ischemic heart disease. *Arch. Intern. Med.* 128:956–960, 1971.

32. Gori, G.B. Diet and cancer. *J. Am. Diet. Assoc.* 71:375–379, 1977.

33. Burkitt, D.P. Large bowel cancer: An epidemiological jigsaw puzzle. *J. Natl. Cancer Inst.* 34:3–6, 1975.

34. Wynder, E.L. Dietary habits and cancer epidemiology. *Cancer* 46:1955–1961, 1979.

35. Wynder, E.L. Dietary factors related to breast cancer. *Cancer* 46:899–904, 1980.

36. Swift, Jonathan. A modest proposal for preventing the children of poor people in Ireland from being a burden to their parents or country; and for making them beneficial to the publick. In Davis, H. (Ed.), *Prose Works of Jonathan Swift*, vol. 12. *Irish Tracts 1728–1733.* Oxford: Blackwell, 1955. Pp. 109–118.

37. McCay, C.M. Effect of restricted feeding upon aging and chronic diseases in rats and dogs. *Am. J. Public Health* 37:521–528, 1947.

38. Ross, M.H. Dietary behavior and longevity. *Nutr. Rev.* 35:257–265, 1977.

39. U.S. Senate. *Dietary Goals for the United States*, 2nd ed. Washington, D.C.: Government Printing Office, December 1977.

40. Recommendations for prevention program in relation to nutrition and cardiovascular disease. Bureau of Nutritional Sciences, Department of National Health and Welfare, Ottawa, Canada, 1977.

41. Weil, W.E. National dietary goals: Are they justified at this time? *Am. J. Dis. Child.* 133:368–370, 1979.

42. Harper, A.E. Dietary goals—a skeptical view. *Am. J. Clin. Nutr.* 31:310–321, 1978.

43. Walker, W.J. Changing United States life-style and declining vascular mortality: Cause or coincidence. *N. Engl. J. Med.* 297:163–165, 1977.

44. Committee on Nutrition, American Academy of Pediatrics. Should milk drinking in children be discouraged? *Pediatrics* 53:576–582, 1974.

45. Ford, C., Callahan, D., Deatrick, D., et al. AHA Committee Report: Nutrition education in the young. A statement for health professionals. *Circulation* 62:918A–912A, 1980.

46. Parcel, G.S. School health education. In Hoekelman, R.A. (Eds.), *Principles of Pediatrics: Health Care for the Young.* New York: McGraw-Hill, 1978.

47. Dahl, L.K. Salt and hypertension. *Am. J. Clin. Nutr.* 25:231–244, 1972.

48. Page, L., Friend, B. The changing United States diet. *Bio-Science* 28:192–197, 1978.

49. Palgi, A. Recommended energy intake according to United States dietary goals. Letter to the editor. *Am. J. Clin. Nutr.* 34:1166–1167, 1981.

50. Goldblatt, P.B., Moore, M.E., Stunkard, A.J. Social factors in obesity. *J.A.M.A.* 192:1039–1044, 1965.

51. Khosla, T., Lowe, C.R. Obesity and smoking habits. *Br. Med. J.* 4:10–13, 1971.

52. Martinez, G., Nalezienski, J.P. 1980 Update: The recent trend in breast-feeding. *Pediatrics* 67:260–263, 1981.

15 Nutrition Education for the Elderly

Mary Darling, M.P.H., R.D.

When discussing nutrition education, it must be assumed that there are resources and opportunities available to help the elderly improve their nutrition. Since attention is frequently centered on protecting the fragile and vulnerable, it is understandable that deterioration in the later years may be the prevailing emphasis. However, nutrition can improve with old age, as can physical fitness. Educators and health care givers need to be sensitive to the diversity among old people and to facilitate the teaching of nutrition. Care should be taken to ensure that the elderly have the instructions or information they need in order to follow directions for a therapeutic diet, to read labels, or to learn how to prepare unfamiliar foods.

This chapter will describe the components of nutrition education, review current recommendations, and discuss two methods of nutrition education: peer teachers and nutrition messages in home-delivered meals. Topics for nutrition education have been identified in previous chapters and will not be discussed here.

Defining Nutrition Education

According to the American Dietetic Association's position paper on the scope and thrust of nutrition education, the objective of nutrition education is to transmit knowledge to consumers about their nutritional needs and the nutritive value of foods in a way that will motivate them to transform this knowledge into eating behavior that promotes health and well-being [1]. According to Esther Peterson, formerly Special Assistant to the President for Consumer Affairs, "Nutrition education is the sum total of the *experience*, *knowledge*, and *skill* possessed by the individual and the family and used to translate health concerns into the act of buying and consuming food" [2]. Godfrey M. Hochbaum, Professor of Health Education and Behavioral Sciences at the University of North Carolina, has stated that nutrition education, no matter how effective, will not have much impact by itself. He points out that educators must coordinate their efforts with lawmakers, regulating agencies, food producers, and food processors over a long period of time in order to make lasting changes in the food culture of the public [3]. Hochbaum has also stated that the nutrition educator must not assume that the public's food selection is motivated by health aspects or that people must learn the concepts and facts that are at the core of the nutritionist's world. Instead, the nutrition educator must assess the underlying factors that determine a target population's present food practices and adapt educational approaches to these factors [4]. Thus the challenge that a nutrition educator faces is bounded by the parameters of knowledge, skills, experience, and underlying factors.

Old people are more variable and more individualistic than any other group in our population [5]. Their health and nutrition knowledge, their methods of food preparation, and their life-styles make each one unique. However, the factors in their social environments that have influenced them—food technology, food laws and regulations, economic conditions—have generated some common life experiences that nutrition educators can recognize in working with older adults.

Assessing the Environment That Influences Eating Habits

People who were born 60 to 80 years ago have lived from a time of wood-burning stoves to microwave ovens, from ice boxes to frozen entrées. The kitchen used to be the only warm room in the house on wintery mornings. Today a kitchen may be a small corner where one person works alone. It is understandable that a widowed elderly woman may discount her own nutritional needs and conclude that there is no one to cook for anymore.

Food prices have soared beyond imagination, and it is difficult for an elderly person to comprehend that nourishing foods are indeed worth the price when he can remember throwing away surplus garden produce or butchering his own meat when he lived on the farm.

The use of food additives, medicated feeds, and pesticides has increased the abundance of our food supply. The science of nutrition has developed during the lifetime of these elderly people. The messages of dietary guidance have been modified, and nutrition education—scientifically based and otherwise—has greater visibility.

Changes have occurred, and the people who have lived through this century are the survivors who have adapted. Although their health or material resources may limit their activities, older adults continue to learn life skills needed for successful aging. However, change for the sake of change is not always necessary. It may be as important to reinforce existing healthful eating habits as it is to try to change them.

Recommendations for Nutrition Education for the Elderly

In 1972 Title VII of the Older Americans Act authorized the Nutrition Program for Older Americans (P.L. 92–258). Among the services offered was nutrition and consumer education. In 1981 it was estimated that 8.4 percent of those 60 years old and older participated in the nutrition program [5]. This act provided incentive for more professionals to be involved in nutrition education, and Title III-c of the amended act continues to authorize this activity.

In 1980 the National Association of Area Agencies on Aging analyzed the nutrition education activities at the nutrition projects for the elderly [6]. Questionnaires were mailed to the 1,032 nutrition service providers, and 496 responded (49%), representing 5,726 meal sites. Ninety-six percent of the meal sites provide nutrition education. Half of the sites provide nutrition education once a month; another 16% provide it twice a month. These activities are provided by registered dietitians or nutritionists (37%), extension home economists (21%), volunteers (21%), and others. Seventy-six percent of the projects interviewed the participants to determine if the nutrition education was beneficial. Of this group, 60% of the responses were positive, 11% were negative, and 29% were indifferent. As a result of this survey, several recommendations were made to the Administration on Aging. Among them were the recommendations to (1) develop a strategy to meet the needs for nutrition education training requested by the providers; (2) provide technical assistance in the development of tools that can be used to evaluate the programs; and (3) develop a clearinghouse for gathering and disseminating instructional materials.

Similar recommendations were made by two other groups. In the report of the 1979 National Conference on Nutrition Education, the task force on low income and elderly populations recommended that the preparation of nutrition educators be strengthened and thorough evaluation of nutrition education programs be required. They stated that the mass media must be a major component of the programs [7]. The other recommendations were from the 1981 Nutrition Education Conference for Older Americans in New York [5]. A series of policy recommendations for both the private and the public sector were developed. These recommendations reiterate: (1) the need for a national policy on nutrition education with special emphasis on target groups such as the aged; (2) that older people must be involved in the planning strategies; (3) that nutrition professionals should guide the design, implementation, and evaluation of education policies and programs; (4) that the federal government should encourage the development of education programs through continued financing of nutrition research and training programs; and (5) that the print and electronic mass media should be used.

The state of nutrition education for older adults is changing, and progress is being made as professionals collaborate. Printed materials are available for the professional as well as the older adult from both the government and the private sector. Computer programs and cable television will become sources of nutrition information in the future. The need to evaluate the effectiveness of such methods will continue. The status of two methods is presented in the following section.

Examples of Nutrition Education Methods

Peer Teachers

The assumption that older people can teach their peers about nutrition appeals to nutrition educators because it multiplies their outreach and involves the older participant in the process. The Administration on Aging and the Center for Disease Control are cooperating in an effort to test and evaluate this idea. The completion date of the project was September 1981 [8].

In 1979 a survey of 459 older Minnesotans was performed to gather information about their ideas on methods of nutrition education, including teaching others. The survey also questioned them on their attitudes about changing eating habits. Adult educators theorize that adults learn more if they are actively involved. When asked to indicate their preferences (Table 15-1), the respondents indicated that they preferred the old classroom model or passive methods of teaching, such as listening to a speaker, reading books or articles, or watching films or slides. Except in the case of trying recipes, active methods were less interesting to them. They were also asked to indicate where they had learned the most about nutrition, by checking three sources from a list of nine items (Table 15-2). "Mother" was checked the most frequently (24% of responses), with "doctor," "magazines," "family," and "dietitian" receiving between 17% and 11% of the responses. Men checked "family" (18.0%) more frequently than women (8.4%), presumably reflecting their spouses' influence. Women checked "magazines" (14.1%) more frequently

Table 15–1
Percentage of Older Adults Indicating Interest in Active and Passive Methods of Nutrition Education

Type of Method	*Interest (%)*	*No Interest (%)*	*No Reply (%)*
Passive			
Listen to speaker	71	21	7
Read books / articles	68	24	7
See film or slides	66	27	7
Active			
Try recipes for 1 or 2	72	23	5
Discussion groups	48	42	10
Teach school-age children	37	54	8
Talk privately about diet	36	56	8
Prepare bulletin board	34	57	9
Help plan menus	31	54	15
Teach peers	25	65	10

Source: M. Darling, unpublished data from a 1979 survey.

Table 15-2
Older Adults' Indication of Sources of Nutrition Information in Their Past

Source	*Percentage of Responses*
Your mother	24
Doctor	17
Magazines	13
Family	11
Dietitian	11
Trial and error	8
School	5
Television	5
Other	4

Source: M. Darling, unpublished data from a 1979 survey.

than men (9.7%). In the last category of "other," Weight Watchers, Inc., was written in by four people.

To identify older adults who might be interested in peer education, it was thought that it would be helpful to know if the subjects had had previous experience as volunteer teachers or leaders. The answer to this question was then compared to their indication of interest in teaching nutrition education to their peers or to school-age children. The results (Table 15-3) indicate that the group with previous experience tended to be more interested (16% and 20%) than those without experience (12% and 16%). If a professional educator is recruiting volunteer teachers from among the elderly, previous experience may be of some help in identifying interested parties. However, the search for volunteer peer educators will require perseverance, as it does in recruiting volunteers from any age group.

At the same time that the survey was being conducted, we piloted a nutrition education training project (six sessions in four weeks) for 11 volunteers in a south central Minnesota community. Most of the volunteers were middle-aged women working with the elderly in housing facilities, nutrition meal sites, or senior centers. After 12 hours of training, they agreed to spend 12 hours teaching the elderly about nutrition. In the next four months they made 1,800 contacts in their community. This demonstrates the remarkable multiplier effect of this method, and it does not count the people who read the posters in laundry rooms or the articles in newspapers. One disadvantage of this method, however, is that the professional must relinquish the control of the nutrition information and take the risk that a less qualified person might make a mistake and give out inaccurate information. In the project's evaluation session, one of the older volunteers said that she knew that her peers often felt that a young professional had not lived long enough to really be an

Table 15-3
A Study of Older Adults' Interest in Teaching Others Compared with Their Previous Experience as Volunteer Teachers

Activity and Interest	*Volunteer Experience (%)*[a]	*No Volunteer Experience (%)*[b]
Teaching nutrition to peers		
Interested	16	12
Not interested	33	37
Teaching school-age children how to cook, bake, or garden		
Interested	20	16
Not interested	30	33

Source: M. Darling, unpublished data from a 1979 survey.
[a]n = 179.
[b]n = 240.

authority. Yet she felt that peers did not regard her as an expert either; she was just one of them.

The peer support model was used as a framework for 19 workshops in three locations conducted by the Turner Geriatric Clinic in Ann Arbor, Michigan [9]. Two of the workshops were on money management and nutrition. In this series, peer counselors identified the topics and speakers and facilitated the discussion groups and evaluation. They were available to follow up on specific needs that were identified in their communities. The use of the peer counselors and the preparation of the speakers resulted in a series of stimulating sessions. The sessions on money management and nutrition provided new information to 97% of the participants. Ninety-three percent felt that the information was practical. In a follow-up telephone interview two to three weeks after the workshop, it was found that 13% had practiced a suggested technique, 46% had changed a routine or habits, and 78% said that they had received information they would use in the future.

It has been demonstrated that peer teacher-counselors can multiply the outreach of professional nutrition educators, and they can improve the effectiveness of the education program. However, it requires considerable effort to identify these individuals.

Nutrition Messages in Home-Delivered Meals

Another method of nutrition education that is frequently viewed as having potential is the network of home-delivered meals. To assess the nutrition knowledge of people who receive such meals, 27 clients were interviewed.

They were asked to respond to 18 food and nutrition words to determine their ability to discuss how the item affected their health. The food items were *milk, vegetables, meat, ice cream, eggs, fruits,* and *oranges*. Nutritional terms included *nutrients, vitamin C, calories, calcium, cholesterol, protein, fat, vitamin A*, and *enriched* or *enrichment*. Other words were *salt* and *bran*. The participants were asked to describe how the items affected their health, and one minute was allowed for each response. The replies were put in three categories: (1) general health response, (2) nutrient knowledge, and (3) other responses. Of the 27 people interviewed, between 10 and 17 responded to each item.

In the first category of health-related responses, the comments included phrases like "I feel better, stronger" or "I feel good." Responses to the words *salt, cholesterol,* and *fat* included "Not good for me, a little is needed" and "Can't use." The word *milk* brought the most responses, with 12 people identifying milk with their general health. Two people associated milk with bones. Only one response identified a nutrient found in milk; calcium was named.

The responses were often stated in terms of frequency of consumption, such as necessary to have every day, every night, or three or four times a week; too much or not enough. The concepts of balance, moderation, and a routine pattern of eating were frequently referred to as being desirable. Meat and fruit were identified the most frequently as being needed daily.

The second category of responses described the ability of the subjects to name the common nutrients associated with a food. The responses were very limited. The word *cholesterol* generated eight responses, with people mentioning eggs (four), meat (three), and margarine (one). Except for the relationship between calcium, bones, and milk mentioned by one person, the subjects did not associate the role of a food item's nutrients with their health.

There was very little inaccurate information. Most people either did not respond or said they did not know.

As a result of this work, we are piloting a set of cards that are being enclosed with the home-delivered meal to determine whether the participants are aware of the cards and the nutrition information.

Because of their limited usable vocabulary concerning nutrition, the need to adapt nutrition education for older adults is evident. The method of reaching them is a dilemma. It is true that 75 to 80 years of lifelong eating habits must be respected. However, people of all ages benefit from good nutrition, and they should not be cut off from opportunities to learn.

Summary

Nutrition education for older adults presents many challenges. It is agreed that good nutrition is important for elderly people, but efficient and effective methods of nutrition education need to be identified. The knowledge, skills, experience, and underlying aspects of the target population must be considered. Peer teachers and messages in home-delivered meals are two methods that are being used and evaluated.

References

1. Position paper on the scope and thrust of nutrition education. *J. Am. Diet. Assoc.* 72:302–305, 1978.

2. Peterson, E. Making nutrition education really work. *J. Nutr. Educ.* 12 (Suppl.):92–93, 1980.

3. Hochbaum, G.M. Strategies and their rationale for changing people's eating habits. *J. Nutr. Educ.* 13 (Suppl.):S59–S63, 1981.

4. Hochbaum, G.M. Human behavior and nutrition education. *Nutrition News* (National Dairy Council), vol. 40, no. 1, 1977, pp. 1, 4.

5. Posner, B. Nutrition education for older Americans: National policy recommendations. *J. Am. Diet. Assoc.* 80L455–458, 1982.

6. Analysis of nutrition education activities at nutrition projects for the elderly. The National Association of Area Agencies on Aging, Washington, D.C., 1980.

7. Brun, J.K., Clancy, K.L. Low income and elderly populations: Task force report. *J. Nutr. Educ.* 12 (Suppl.):128–130, 1980.

8. Greene, J.M. Coordination of Older Americans Act programs. *J. Am. Diet. Assoc.* 78:617–620, 1981.

9. Campbell, R., Chenoweth, B. Health education as a basis for social support. *Gerontologist* 21:619–627, 1981.

16 Legislation Affecting the Nutritional Status of the Elderly

Paul A. Kerschner, Ph.D.
Barbara K. Herzog, Ph.D.

Nutritional Status of the Elderly

Current Status

Let us begin on a positive note. Robert Butler, director of the National Institute on Aging, and others have made the point about how much better off the elderly are now than they were in the last century. Among the factors Dr. Butler points to is the combating of infectious and nutrition-related disease. As we know all too well, this victory has turned the field over to chronic degenerative disease, but we should not lose sight of the fact that this represents major progress and a major extension of life for the U.S. population.

Does this mean that the average older person is consuming an adequately balanced nutritious diet every day? Unfortunately, this is not the case. For example, survey data presented to the 1981 White House Conference on Aging indicated that about two-thirds of the older Americans who were questioned reported daily eating of three meals that were not adequately balanced [1]. For example, only 1 percent eat the prescribed four servings of fruit or vegetables. Nearly half reported only one serving. Only one daily serving of bread or cereals was reported by 47 percent, and only a third eat two servings a day of meat and other proteins. Only 19 percent of those on food stamps eat this recommended amount. Only 31 percent consume at least two daily servings of dairy foods, which are entirely skipped by 16 percent of those on food stamps [2].

Not surprisingly, research indicates that the nutritional status of blacks and other minorities is worse than that of nonminorities [3], due in large part at least to their lower average income. Food in black neighborhoods tends to be priced higher than food in white neighborhoods, and a lack of mobility also results in higher food costs for blacks.

Contributory Factors

There are a multiplicity of factors that have an effect on the dietary intake of the elderly. We will recount these only briefly, because many of them are similar to the factors affecting the diet of the population of all ages. As usual, however, there are a few unique factors.

Income. According to a 1979 report [4], households headed by persons 65 years of age and over accounted for 20 percent of all U.S. households. Yet these households accounted for less than 11 percent of all household income and only about 13 percent of all the money spent for food [4]. The same households, according to U.S government data, accounted for about 14 percent of all at-home food purchases but only about 9 percent of expenditures on away-from-home eating. We will explore this further in a subsequent section, but suffice it to say here that the nutritional difficulties of the elderly are not the result of overdependence on fast food.

Mental Health and Motivation. It is clear that loneliness, grief, apathy, or confusion may play a major role in how much and what an elderly person consumes, even if that person has sufficient income. One need only think of the stereotypic but frequently accurate image of the elderly widow surviving on tea and toast to appreciate the particular importance of the psychological status of the elderly person.

Dentition. Another factor particularly important to the nutritional status of the elderly person is the condition of his or her teeth or dentures. The point is obvious but not appreciated by the funders of Medicare.

Transportation. To the surprise of government officials, transportation turned out to be the "sleeper" issue of both the 1971 and 1981 White House Conferences on Aging. It should have surprised no one to find out that elderly people feel this is one of their major problems, and clearly it affects their ability to get to and from stores to make their food purchases. High bulk and fresh items are often sacrificed by those who cannot easily get to stores or carry home their packages. A related point is the condition of the older person's feet. Again this is an obvious point but one that tends to be overlooked, often by physicians as well as Medicare.

Neighborhood Crime. A fifth factor affecting nutritional status is the presence or absence of serious crime in an older person's neighborhood.

Nutrition Education. As with younger people, knowledge of good nutrition plays a role with the elderly, particularly among lower-income individuals.

Medications. Drug use, including over-the-counter drugs, also plays a role with the elderly just as it does with younger people. However, in older people this role is heightened because of their increased consumption of various medications, including both over-the-counter drugs such as mineral oil laxatives that interfere with absorption of fat-soluble vitamins, and prescription drugs that interfere with vitamin B_{12} and folic acid.

Legislation Directly or Indirectly Affecting the Status of the Elderly

Social Security and Supplemental Security Income

It would be misleading to limit a discussion about legislation affecting the nutritional status of the elderly to those programs such as food stamps or meals-on-wheels that provide food directly. Such programs are very important, but together they affect a relatively small percentage of the elderly. The discussion more properly begins with the income programs that affect the food budget of most of the nation's elderly—Social Security plus its welfare supplement, SSI, or Supplemental Security Income.

Thirty-eight percent of the income of older people is from Social Security. For many it is the only income they have; other sources are public and private pensions (16%), earnings (23%), asset income (19%), and nonspecified other income (4%) [5]. The average Social Security monthly check for an individual is $549 [6]. Given the little-appreciated fact that the elderly are currently paying about three-fifths of their health care expenses out of their own pocket, those people depending on Social Security alone have some real choices to make when they go to the grocery store about how many fresh oranges they are going to buy.

The American Association for Retired Persons (AARP) has fought long and hard to retain existing Social Security benefits, particularly the Social Security cost-of-living increases that keep recipients up with inflation. We have also been working hard to support SSI, which is equally if not more vulnerable to cuts, since this is a program for the poor who are not noted for their eloquent letters to Congressmen. A little-known fact is that in most states SSI currently does not even provide a poverty-level income. The poverty level is currently set at $4,680 for an individual and $6,220 for a couple [7], and AARP's long-held position is that SSI should be set at 25 percent above the poverty level. But realistically, we are fighting to retain what is currently on the books rather than trying for increases that could allow the poor to eat a little better. For the 15 percent of the elderly who are below the poverty line, "heat or eat" is sometimes the grim choice to be faced.

Let us look at the amounts allocated for food in both the Bureau of Labor Statistics (BLS) intermediate budget and the poverty-level budget. In the BLS intermediate budget for a retired couple in 1980, the amount allocated for food for a retired couple with an income of $9,400 per year was $53 per week per couple [8]. This is quite a modest figure, but a careful couple could certainly eat nutritiously at this level. Consider, however, the food budget contemplated for a retired couple right at the poverty line. The food budget contemplated at the poverty line was only $28 per week in 1979, and a bit more today [9]. Note that this figure is for the couple, not for each person. Even this $28 in an unrealistically high estimate, since actual average medical expenses are considerably higher than what is contemplated in the poverty budget, and thus less money, in fact, is left for food.

Now consider the fact that over 15 percent of the elderly (about 4 million people) are *below* the poverty line, and many millions more are just barely above it—and these numbers have increased over the past several years. These people are not likely to be eating a balanced, nutritious diet, even if they are lucky enough to have some teeth or dentures that don't hurt, and transportation to a store. Are they likely to say so in the physician's consulting room? Perhaps they will, if you ask them directly, but probably not: we find that older people by and large are not likely to complain about their economic status.

Food Stamps

The food stamp program provides assistance to at least 2.026 million elderly persons aged 60 and older, according to most recent data [10]. Participation has been increasing since the food stamp purchase requirement was removed. Between November 1978 and November 1979, for example, the number of elderly persons receiving food stamps increased by 42 percent, whereas participation among the nonelderly increased by only 26 percent [10].

Older Americans Act Title III Nutrition Program

One of the best known social programs in America today is the meals-on-wheels program, with its catchy title and almost undisputed utility. This program is operated through the Older Americans Act Title III, which also provides funding for the congregate meals programs that take place around the country. The Department of Agriculture contributes some food as well as one-quarter of the funding. The congregate meals programs are considered nutrition programs, but one needs to remember that this is nutrition in a very broad sense, and it includes opportunities for socialization and access to information as well. One of the program's founders, Bernard Nash, former director of the AARP, reminded us recently that from the program's very inception, socialization was considered just as important as the provision of food (personal communication). The funding for these two programs is a real drop in the budgetary bucket—just over $583 million in 1982, and one-quarter of this is from nonfederal sources. Like other social service programs, this one has been cut back and will be held to 1982 levels in 1983, according to reports from Washington.

Medicare and Lack of Coverage for Dental and Foot Care

The point is obvious, and we will not belabor it. If a person's dentures hurt with every bite, he or she does not eat a very balanced diet, and if his toenails are ingrown, he or she goes to the store less frequently and probably spends less time walking. The American Association of Retired Persons has urged for years that dental and foot care be included in Medicare coverage. Until they are, there will continue to be serious detriments to the preconditions for good nutrition.

Mandatory Retirement and the Age Discrimination in Employment Act

Legislation passed several years ago makes it illegal, as a general rule, to forcibly retire an individual based on his or her age up to the age of 70 [11]. Most people should not be forced to retire until age 70, but in practice mandatory retirement still frequently occurs. One reason is that the Age Discrimination in Employment Act (ADEA) is not enforced well at the federal level because of budgetary staffing limitations. Moreover, many people are not aware of their rights under the law.

Another difficulty is that sometimes it is hard to tell whether a person is being fired because of his or her age or because of other reasons such as declining performance. In these cases individuals may be deterred from bringing suit because of their uncertainty as to cause—or the possibility of losing an expensive case in a situation that is not clear-cut.

The American Association of Retired Persons has strongly supported tough enforcement of ADEA, as well as legislation abolishing mandatory retirement. Critics have cited the possibility of a massive flood of older people hanging on to their jobs and clogging the advancement pipeline. In fact, it is interesting to note that the Department of Labor estimates that by 1985, as a result of the legislation raising the age to 70, only about an additional 250,000 workers will be on the job [11].

The Association believes strongly in options—that the individual should have a choice, assuming he or she is doing a competent job, of retiring or not retiring. Those who want to stay on and retain the more adequate income should be able to do so, but they should not be forced to do so through legislation raising the age of Social Security benefit eligibility to 68. The Association's position is that there should be strong incentives to induce older people to keep on working and earning—and, not incidentally, to keep paying taxes. But we do not want to force a burned-out steel worker to continue to age 68. The main incentives to continued work that we favor are abolishing the Social Security earnings limitation and raising the amount of Social Security benefits one receives if one postpones retirement to an actuarially fair amount. Currently, a person begins to lose Social Security benefits after he or she has earned $6,000. And currently, a person receives only a 3-percent increment in benefits for each year he or she postpones retirement. This should be raised to an actuarially accurate figure, or about 9 percent per year.

If these steps are taken, we believe many individuals will be better off because of the increased income from work that they will retain. Lest one think that this will benefit only the upper-middle class, let us point out some salient survey data: According to a 1974 Harris poll [1], those retirees who *most* wanted to have continued work were those making less than $5,000 per year. We do not have more recent data on that, but given inflation and poor economic conditions, the desire to work is not likely to have decreased.

What is likely to happen legislatively in the future? We are optimistic concerning the earnings limitation, and concerning at least *some* increase in the amount of increase in Social Security as a result of delaying retirement. We are less optimistic about the abolition of mandatory retirement. In a recent speech President Reagan stated he favored changing the laws so that mandatory retirement at any age would be illegal. We now note reports in the news media, however, that pressure from business leaders has led him to change his mind. Thus we are not anticipating any further legislation from this Administration regarding mandatory retirement, except, possibly, to weaken the ADEA protection.

Medicaid and Nursing Home Inspections

The level of Medicaid payments to nursing homes in most states is relatively low—lower than the average bill in the average nursing home. The result is not surprising: in general (and there are many specific exceptions), the overall level and quality of care in Medicaid nursing homes are lower than in homes where there are relatively few Medicaid patients. It is our impression, although we have no data to back this up, that it follows that the diet provided in Medicaid homes is generally inferior to that in non-Medicaid homes—again with many exceptions.

At the moment, the Department of Health and Human Services is embroiled in a controversy about how much to cut back the nursing home regulations and, in particular, about the required number of inspections for Medicare-certified institutions. Although the debate does not revolve around nutrition, it seems to me that the substantial cutbacks that are being proposed in the frequency of inspections are likely to have a depressing influence on the quality of the food.

Nutrition Programs for the Nation's Future Elderly: Children

Although the subject of this chapter is the elderly, we would be remiss if we did not mention the AARP's concern over the fate of legislation affecting the nation's future elderly. In fact, nutrition programs for children are in big trouble—more trouble even than programs for the elderly. Unlike AARP's articulate and enthusiastic members, children do not write letters, do not march, and above all, do not vote. The result has been that they, like the poor, have been relatively easy targets for budget cuts. We will just mention a few of the programs that have suffered severely in the last several years. The best known of these is the WIC, or Women, Infants, and Children, program. Another is the school lunch program and its summer counterpart, the summer feeding program. The use of catsup as a vegetable should have warned us of what was to come, but we forget these warnings all too soon. Third, the special milk program and the food stamp program for children have also been sharply cut back. Finally, the nutrition education and training program, an innovative and, in my view, cost-beneficial program started in 1977, will receive no more funding by 1983. This program formerly gave each state 50 cents per school child for education about *why* they should eat certain foods and go easy on certain others, and used the school lunch program as a laboratory. Given the impact of television advertising on the nation's children, 50 cents seems little enough to try to build some countervailing pressures against the high-cholesterol, high-sugar diets toward which our market system is propelling children.

In sum, let me emphasize that we at AARP are aware of the cumulative effect of nutrition over the years and are thus disturbed that what little money had been set aside to improve children's nutritional status is now being cut away.

Government Regulations and Reports

The Federal Trade Commission and the Food and Drug Administration

In line with the ideological predisposition of its Reagan-appointed chairman and senior staff, the Federal Trade Commission (FTC) is abandoning the use of rule making rather than case-by-case enforcement as a means of establishing industry-wide uniform standards of marketplace behavior. Food advertising rules will be no exception to this retreat. The head of the Bureau of Consumer Protection at the FTC recently recommended to the full commission that the commission drop the proposed food rule, which would have governed a variety of claims concerning cholesterol and other matters of health significance.

The Food and Drug Administration (FDA), however, recently proposed a rule concerning labeling with sodium information which should, if adopted, lead to more useful information labeling concerning sodium content.

National Academy of Sciences Reports

In June 1982 the National Academy of Sciences released a report calling for a sharp cutback in the nation's consumption of fatty meat, butter, whole milk, alcohol, and salt- or smoked-cured meats. It also urged an increase in the consumption of fruits, vegetables, and whole-grain bread or cereals [12]. That this is needed is not news to any of us, but it is heartening that the government is increasingly willing to take a stand on controversial issues and to make recommendations opposed by significant segments of the U.S. food industry.

Local Regulations on Supermarket Unit Pricing

Supermarkets are increasingly moving away from marking each individual item. We believe that this is an unfortunate trend which makes it more difficult to do comparison shopping and increases the problems for older people in intelligent purchase of foodstuffs. Regulations such as these must be carefully watched as part of our effort to maintain or improve the nutritional status of the nation's older population.

Prospects for the Future

Perhaps because of the climate in Washington these days and the unprecedented difficulties Congress is having in producing a budget, we are not very optimistic about any improvement in the nutritional status of the elderly as a result of improved legislation. We will be lucky to hang on to what we have, at least in the next few years. We are particularly concerned that the budget cuts are having the heaviest impact on the poor—elderly, middle-aged, and children—who are the least vocal and the least able to persuade Congress and the Administration that their support matters.

We may do a bit better in the area of consumer education. Currently we are riding a wave of "self-help," particularly among middle- and upper-income groups. People want to change and have shown themselves actually willing to change their smoking and eating habits and to try to influence their health and longevity. According to a recent Harvard University study of physicians' smoking and eating habits, even physicians seem to have changed.

Newspapers, magazines, and television all seem more interested in prevention as well, and we hope that we can encourage them to go further in the direction of offering nutrition education to the public.

What Physicians and Other Health Professionals Can Do

We strongly suspect that a good deal of malnutrition among the elderly is not being detected in the physician's office. As clinicians, most physicians and other health professionals probably could be more careful to ensure that their patients are not, in fact, suffering from nutritional deficiencies. In a 1980 issue of the *Journal of the American Medical Association* [13], a discussion of so-called senility indicated that there are more than 100 reversible disorders that can mimic organic brain syndromes, including vitamin B deficiencies. Are physicians doing everything they can to ensure that patients they send to nursing homes or those who are already there and confused do not suffer from nutritional deficiencies?

What about osteoporosis? Are we doing all we can to prevent this condition, which immobilizes and often kills so many older women through hip fractures? Physicians should encourage whatever combination of exercise, calcium intake, and vitamin D intake seems indicated in order to retard osteoporosis.

Obtaining nutritional information can be a time-consuming task. If physicians are not already doing this, they could have their patients fill out questionnaires, or their receptionists or even volunteers could obtain nutritional information on their patients. At AARP we have embarked on a health advocacy program. We are training volunteers to work with other older people to improve their knowledge of and practices concerning their health, and nutrition is an important part of this effort.

Summary

Infection and nutrition-related diseases as causes of major disability in the elderly have been largely supplanted by chronic degenerative diseases. Although this represents major progress and an extension of life for the U.S.

population, significant subsets of the elderly population remain undernourished. Blacks and other minorities fare worse than others in this regard.

In the young and elderly populations, in general, the ultimate influences on nutrition are several, and dietary problems may develop gradually over many years. Social and medical factors such as mental and emotional problems, lack of transportation, crime in neighborhoods, deficient nutrition education, poor dentition or foot care, and chronic use of medication may all lead, directly or indirectly, to malnutrition. Legislation and government programs strongly influence the availability of food for the young and the elderly. Solutions to the problems of nutrition will require a coordinated effort on the part of consumers, health professionals, and government bodies. The AARP has embarked on a health advocacy program, and nutritional education is an important part of this effort.

References

1. Allan, C., Brotman, H. (Eds.). *Chartbook on Aging in America.* The 1981 White House Conference on Aging (C.D. Armitage, chairman). Washington, D.C.: Government Printing Office, 1981.

2. Brunelle, C. *The Gray Paper.* A Presentation to the 1981 White House Conference on Aging. Rye, N.Y.: ITT Continental Baking, 1981.

3. Baeley, F.E., Walker, M.L. Socio-economic factors and their effects on the nutrition and dietary habits of the black aged. *J. Gerontol. Nursing* 8:203–207, 1982.

4. Gallo, A.E., Boehm, W.T., LeBovit, C. *Food Expenditure Patterns and Assistance.* Agricultural Economic Report no. 426, U.S. Department of Agriculture. Washington, D.C.: Government Printing Office, 1979.

5. U.S. Social Security Administration. *Income and Resources of the Aged, 1978.* Washington, D.C.: Government Printing Office, 1982.

6. U.S. Social Security Administration. *Social Security Bulletin Annual Statistical Supplement, 1980.* Washington, D.C.: Government Printing Office, 1980.

7. H.H.S. raises poverty guidelines by ten percent. *The Older American Reports*, vol. 6, no. 15, p. 3, April 1982.

8. U.S. Bureau of the Census. Current Population Reports, Series P-60, no. 133. Characteristics of the population below the poverty level, 1980. Washington, D.C.: Government Printing Office, 1982.

9. Smeeding, T.R. *Alternative Methods for Valuing Selected In-Kind Transfer Benefits and Measuring Their Effect on Poverty.* U.S. Bureau of the Census Technical Paper no. 50, C3.212. Washington, D.C.: Government Printing Office, 1982.

10. U.S. Congress, Senate Special Committee on Aging. Developments in aging. A report of the Special Committee on Aging. U.S. Senate, 97th Congress, Second Session, 1981.

11. U.S. Congress. Age Discrimination in Employment Act and Amendments of 1978. U.S. Code vol. 29, p. 621, P.L. 95–256, April 6, 1978, U.S. Statutes vol. 92, p. 189. Washington, D.C.: Government Printing Office, 1978.

12. Cohn, V. Reshaping the nation's diet. *Washington Post*, June 17, 1982, p. A1.

13. National Institute on Aging Consensus Task Force. Senility reconsidered: Treatment possibilities for mental impairment in the elderly. *J.A.M.A.* 244:259–263, 1980.

17 National Food Resources, Policies, and Responsibilities: An Appraisal

William F. Hueg, Jr., Ph.D.

My purpose in this chapter is to call attention to the agricultural system in the United States, which is clearly the legacy of the land-grant university. Agriculture was not always as we know it in the United States today. We need not travel too far in the world to see what our agriculture was like 20 and 50 years ago and, after a relatively brief plane ride, to see the agriculture of 2,000 years ago and more.

Our agriculture, which is about 12,000 to 15,000 years old, had very humble beginnings. It was probably invented by women out of their frustration and dissatisfaction with the inability of their men to provide adequately for the growing human family. There are those who still argue whether agriculture is a science. It is true that agriculture is both art and science, but I would suggest that agriculture is the mother science.

It was not until agriculture had improved to the point that it was possible to produce a food surplus over the immediate needs of the cultivators that organized knowledge (science) was possible. Agriculture has been said to be the science that allows life as we know it to flourish, and it may well be that before the century is over, judgment of the success of science as a whole will rest on the success or failure of agriculture.

The social impact of agricultural science, whether it was the early domestication of plants and animals, the innovation of rotations and mixed farming in Europe, the invention of the binder-reaper, the application of the Mendelian principles to breeding and artificial selection, the green revolution of more modern times, or the future impact of genetic engineering and molecular biology, cannot be in doubt. The scientific knowledge that created these innovations gave rise to cities, to industry, to modern class society. It fed armies, nurtured scholars and artists, and transformed the social and political structure of the world. These ideas are nicely summarized in a quotation from Jonathan Swift's *Gulliver's Travels*: "And he gave it for his opinion that whoever could make two ears of corn or two blades of grass to grow upon a spot of ground where only one grew before would deserve better of mankind and do more essential service to his country than a whole race of politicians put together" [1]. This quotation and the preceding comments truly place agriculture in the realm of science in action.

U.S. Agriculture: A Productive Giant

American agriculture is the envy of the world. It is a low-cost and efficient agriculture. It produces enormous and increasing quantities of food and fiber at prices and costs that are among the lowest in the world. It can be calculated that today, somewhat fewer than 3.5 million workers provide almost all the food for 220 million Americans, and we still export the output of almost 40 percent of the total crop land of our country. The United States is the world's largest exporter of agricultural products. Our share of the world's export of major farm products makes impressive statistics: wheat, 40 percent; feed grain, 72 percent; soybeans, 80 percent; tobacco, 20 percent; cotton, 30 percent. The United States accounts for nearly 20 percent of the total value of world agricultural exports. In 1981 we exported $44 billion worth of agricultural products, while importing just $16 billion for an enormous $28 billion net surplus of agricultural trade. The agricultural economies of the developing world stand in stark contrast. It is hard to believe that as recently as 1963 we were a net importer of agricultural products.

One of the great dilemmas facing U.S. agriculture today is that it is almost too successful and has literally been taken for granted by the decision makers and citizens of this country. While the United States is generally believed to be in a recession, it is probably true that agriculture is already in a depression. In my own state of Minnesota, the net income of farmers has diminished each year in the recent five-year period, in spite of "bin-busting" yields of crops and ever more efficient yields of livestock products. The major dilemma facing the farmer is one of cash flow in an industry which has increasingly substituted capital for labor over the past 30 years, and which has become increasingly dependent on outside sources for production inputs in order to achieve the large productivity of which we boast.

U.S. agriculture is still relatively independent in terms of individual decision making by the entrepreneurial American farmer, but increasingly this freedom of choice is being circumscribed by others because of a growing dependence on outside capital and other inputs and on world markets. The American farmer cannot be described with one word but only with combinations, such as businessman, mechanic, husbandman, scientist, marketer, and salesman. Most farmers do not describe themselves in this way.

U.S. agriculture is not perfect. Over the last two decades we have seen a decline in numbers of farms, an increasing difficulty in entering farming, and the concentration of agribusiness, all of which are of concern to society. At one time, U.S. agriculture was very independent and isolationist. Today it has become highly interdependent and is far from isolationist in its influence on world events, as well as in its contributions to the developed and developing world. If it had not been for the success of U.S. agriculture, the world and not just the United States would be facing even greater difficulties than it currently is. There are great challenges for the future. It is the challenge of science at all levels to assure that we have an adequately to well-fed population. The enormity of this challenge must be considered in light of events as they happen [2]:

In the last 60 seconds,

164 people have been added to the world population; about 33 (one-fifth) of these will be fed by the United States, which has 5 percent of the world population.

In the last 60 seconds,

annual world demand for agricultural products has increased by:

1,240 bushels of coarse grains (as corn) (this is 12 acres at 100 bushels per acre),
690 bushels of wheat,
690 bushels of rice,
200 bushels of oilseeds (as soybeans),
4,050 pounds of beef (6 steers),
3,840 pounds of pork (23 hogs),
2,140 pounds of poultry (765 chickens),
1,150 pounds of cotten (2.4 bales),
490 pounds of mutton/lamb (15 sheep).

Role of the Land-Grant University in U.S. Agriculture

The success of U.S. agriculture is relatively recent in the historical perspective. Agriculture over the two hundred years of the nation has had problems of poverty more often than prosperity. For the first hundred years of our history, in fact until as late as 1880, agricultural exports accounted for some 80 percent of total U.S. exports. We should remember that the Revolutionary War was basically a war over the conduct of agricultural trade.

Between 1880 and 1970, the United States lost its place as a major exporter of agricultural products. In 1972 the export surplus was only $2 billion; in 1981, only 10 years later, that export surplus was $28 billion. We will have great difficulty holding this record level of surplus export, however, because of weak prices and even weaker world markets. For a long period, between 1889 and 1919, the total productivity of U.S. agriculture only increased at an annual rate of 0.02 percent. The increase in output during this period was nearly matched by an equivalent increase in input of land, labor, and machinery. This situation was no different from that being faced by agriculture in developing countries today. The reasons for the transformation of U.S. agriculture that occurred in this century are multiple and complex, but they are clearly related to the application of agricultural science through the land-grant university system. Farm population did not begin to decline until

1910, and the number of farms did not decline until the 1930s. It was the willingness of farmers and industry to capitalize on the public investment in research and education that brought about this transformation.

The concept of agricultural and mechanical colleges began to take shape in the 1850s. The goal was to establish a college in each state funded by grants of federal land. The purpose was to teach the children of mechanics, artisans, and farmers. The first land-grant bill was vetoed by President Buchanan in 1861, but the following year the newly elected Abraham Lincoln, needing support of the states leaning to the South, signed a new bill, the Morrill Act, on July 2, 1862. Speaking on the twenty-fifth anniversary of the land-grant act, Justin Morrill said, "The land-grant colleges were founded on the idea that a higher and broader education should be placed in every state within the reach of those whose destiny assigned them to or may have the courage to choose industrial vocations where the wealth of nations is produced" [3]. It was in 1887 with the passage of the Hatch Act that states began to have the opportunity to receive federal funding for the support of research, and in 1914 the Smith-Lever Act provided that same opportunity for establishing extension activities. The developments were slow, but the process has evolved into the modern land-grant university with strong commitments to teaching, research, and extension. This was truly an institutional revolution.

In those early years there was little agricultural knowledge to teach, and that which was available was borrowed from Europe and taught primarily by professors of botany or chemistry. It was really not until the 1930s that such science-based innovations as hybrid corn and chemical fertilizers started the agricultural revolution that powered the United States' emergence from the Great Depression, assisted in the control of the dust bowl, supported a war effort in World War II, fed a starved and crippled Europe and Japan after the war, and led to the emergence of today's agriculture and its contribution to world food supplies.

This system in the land-grant universitites, in the private universities that conduct agricultural research, teaching, and extension, and in the private sector is truly being challenged. The history of the next 20 years will tell whether we have appropriately adjusted and accepted the responsibilities for today and tomorrow or whether we are willing to rest on the laurels of a past and present glory.

Challenge of the 1980s

The foregoing discussion is all part of the history that has set the stage for the development of the agricultural system as we know it. Agriculture in both the United States and the world is in a depression. This has come about for many reasons, but primarily it is one of a surplus of very inelastic demand commodities, grains in particular. In 1973, when the world had food scares, we were short in these inelastic demand commodities. These violent swings and roller-coaster effects will probably continue to characterize world agriculture through the 1980s.

Our own government has no clear policy on market development or on what it wants the U.S. farmer and the agricultural system to do. Three major trade embargoes over the last decade have moved us from being a primary supplier of grain to now being a residual supplier. This makes a tremendous difference in how successful we can be in trading with world partners. Recently, the secretaries of state and of defense have been encouraging President Reagan not to sign another round of grain trading arrangements with the Soviet Union. (The previous arrangement ended September 30, 1982.) We should have learned by now, after these unsuccessful embargoes, that such actions only hurt the U.S. farmer and thus the economy and society of the United States, and create more opportunities for other "green belt" nations to market their grain.

With all the furor about trading arrangements and surplus grain supplies, the fact remains that about one-quarter of the world's population is at near-starvation or starvation level. One does not have to go to Third World nations to find people who are malnourished or who are on the low end of the calorie intake scale. A 1982 article by Hulse in *Science* speaks on "Food Science and Nutrition: The Gulf Between Rich and Poor" [4].

Our domestic food stamp programs are in a shambles. We have milk-marketing orders that do not help producers or consumers. We have continuing and seemingly endless arguments about grading standards for livestock, especially beef grades. One branch of the Department of Agriculture is discussing adequate diets for humans at various age levels, while another branch in the same agency is promoting more production of animal products through research and adoption of new and improved practices. We have one federal agency telling us the dangers and hazards of smoking, and another federal agency subsidizing the production of tobacco.

One has to look long and hard to see even a semblance of policy when it comes to food in the United States. Perhaps the great unwritten policy is "cheap and abundant food." The experience of the last ten years would indicate that in the 1980s, food will still be abundant but not necessarily cheap! There are too many external costs that go into the purchase of food today over which there is little control by the primary producer and much less control on the part of the consumer.

Desire to Improve Nutrition

The developing nations want to improve their levels of nutrition. They see what is happening in more affluent parts of the world and ask why they cannot have the same. These may be legitimate goals, but how rapidly they can be achieved and what kinds of pressure they may place on existing food production systems in these countries and in the world have yet to be decided. We must develop programs to upgrade agricultural production and improve storage and marketing systems in these countries and to develop the ancillary industry that is essential for high-level agricultural production. Better control of population goes hand in hand with these programs, and the sooner such efforts get under way, the better for the specific nation and the world.

The People's Republic of China has made conscious efforts to increase the protein intake of its citizens by 1 percent a year, and the Soviet Union has had a similar goal of 5 percent for the last ten years. A decision of this type has been a major factor in some of the expanding grain trading that goes on in the world. Regardless of such goals, it is extremely difficult to overcome U.S. grain embargoes such as the one established because of the Russian action in Afghanistan.

As Americans, we cannot overlook the cultural and ethical issues that deal with improved nutrition and population control. In many parts of the Third World, the agricultural economy is one of barter rather than exchange of money. In the Sehiel, an economy has developed over centuries based on livestock and the food source for protein from milk and blood. There is also the additional factor that livestock is used as part of a dowry in the marriage system, and a man's wealth is shown by the number of livestock, in particular cattle, that he owns. In India sacred animals consume about 30 percent of the crop production. Moreover, it is still difficult to convince an Indian farmer that he should control the size of this family when his religion speaks to the desire of having many children. In fact, the children are the labor force and the insurance for old age.

The Food Delivery System

The agricultural system in the United States includes primary production as well as the input and output industries. Although the U.S. system is not perfect, it is the envy of much of the world, and there are many attempts in developing nations to modify our system to bring about higher levels of success. There has been continued interest in the United States in reducing the per capita consumption of livestock products and shifting more to natural grain products and vegetables. This trend has had a marked impact on the livestock industry, and I believe that during the period of the 1980s, and certainly by the turn of the century, we will see definite changes in the livestock industry. However, we delude ourselves if we think that by changing our consumption habits of livestock products, we will be making more food available for hungry people in the world. The problem still rests with a poorly developed distribution system, so that even with a surplus, too many people will die from starvation or be maimed by malnutrition.

The time is long past for developing nations to look critically at the adequate feeding of their population. This can only occur by the development of a highly productive agricultural system in each of these countries, including an education and research component such as we know in our land-grant universities. This very system, however, is threatened even in the United States by the decreasing levels of support that come from state and federal appropriations.

My reason for bringing in the issue of appropriation is that the science we need so badly to feed a world population that will nearly double in 40 years will require much larger levels of expenditure than the current ones. Essentially, the easy problems have been tackled and solved; we are now moving into those that are more complex, and breaking the secrets held by nature is becoming increasingly difficult. However, science has been the base of the agricultural system, and it is on that base that future progress will be made, but at a faster pace than that of the last 20 years. Even if we succeeded in providing double yields, we would still have committed one-quarter of the world's population to starvation and low levels of nutrition. This is not a happy picture, but it is one that, as Americans and as citizens of a very complex world, we cannot ignore.

The concentration in this symposium has been on improved nutrition in the young and the elderly. This is a critical issue which faces not only the United States but all of the world. How quickly we place this as a high-priority item depends on what we as individual scientists choose to do about it. In addition to performing our research, we must inform decision makers and those who influence decision makers of the critical nature of what we do. The strength of our system of democracy is that each of us is entitled to a point of view. The more advanced and educated that point of view, the better will be the decision. As scientists working in the areas of nutrition, food, and medicine, we sometimes have waited too long before we have become involved in helping to develop solutions. We should seek to become advocates for the research that we do in order to engender higher levels of understanding about this work and its importance for the continuance of a high level of civilization in the world for the decades and centuries ahead.

Summary

The development of the productive U.S. agricultural system came about by a series of well-defined policies of federal, state, and private initiatives over a period from 1862 to the present. This well-established system is now being challenged because of failure to recognize the importance of this integrated system and its changing structure. To ensure adequate food supplies in the world, agricultural systems in developing nations must take higher priority than they do presently. The success or failure of these systems in the remaining years of this decade will dictate the adequacy of food supplies and levels of nutrition for the billions of people who populate the earth. This responsibility needs to be shared by all in the developed world, with higher priority given by governments in developing nations.

References

1. Swift, J. *Gulliver's Travels.* New York: Grolier, 1971.

2. Jaquier, L.L. *Nitrogen and Phosphate Demand/Supply Now and in 1985.* Chicago: The Fertilizer Institute, 1981.

3. Morrill, J.S. *State Aid to the U.S. Land-Grant Colleges.* Address given on behalf of the University of Vermont and the State Agricultural College delivered in the Hall of Representatives, Montpelier, Vermont, October 10, 1888. Burlington, Vt.: Free Press Association, 1888.

4. Hulse, J.H. Food science and nutrition: The gulf between rich and poor. *Science*, vol. 216 no. 4552 (June 18, 1982), pp. 1291–1294.

Discussion

Questions were addressed to the panel of speakers, which consisted of Ms. Darling, Dr. Robinow, Dr. Kerschner, and Dr. Hueg.

The discussion in this session revolved primarily around issues of public policy. These included satisfying the nuritional needs of the young and elderly population and the interaction between farm production and dietary needs or preferences.

The general opinion was expressed that in the United States the average diet of both young and old people is adequate in meeting basic nutritional needs. However, there exist subpopulations whose special circumstances predispose them toward malnutrition. Among the young, this includes children who are not fed breakfast or who live in unstable family situations. Conversely, those of the elderly who are poor, who reside in nursing homes, and who are chronically ill or bedridden require special attention to ensure that they receive adequate nutritional support.

School lunch programs were regarded as fulfilling the basic needs of the young. Nevertheless, certain subgroups are clearly at risk. Although all other groups of U.S. children have shown improved growth in recent decades, Malina and Savaleta [1] have shown that there has been no increase in height or weight among Mexican-Americans.

Communal feeding programs such as school lunches or congregate feeding of the elderly also present good opportunities for socialization and for introducing ancillary support programs, such as for housing and for medical care. The need for such combined activities has been highlighted by several recent surveys that suggest that the elderly poor, when faced with reduced incomes, first reduce their expenditures for food, then for medical care, and finally for housing.

Nutritional support of the free-living, healthy elderly population has been attempted with commodities feeding programs and with the food stamp program. Neither of these has been regarded as satisfactory. In particular, the commodities feeding programs have encountered problems related to distribution and acceptability of food, lack of a strong educational component, and the inherent danger that either feeding is geared to available commodities or food production becomes directed toward desired commodities. In contrast, the food stamp program eliminates the problem of distribution and offers the user a greater variety of choice. The panel suggested that the reported abuses of the food stamp program are frequently exaggerated and have little significance on the cost of the overall program. Nevertheless, the shortcomings of the food stamp program need to be improved, and one of the most important efforts in this direction would be the introduction of a strong educational component.

Nursing home residents are more vulnerable to the effects of poor nutrition because they have so little influence over their own nutrition. Since the goal of nutrition should always be to enhance the quality of life of the individual, care must be taken in the nursing home that the quality and quantity of meals never become so restrictive that food consumption is reduced and appetite and enjoyment are lost. In this light, the suggestion was made to turn over the responsibility for nutritional care from physicians to dietitians and nurses, who are closer to the residents and who have the direct, daily responsibility for the residents' care.

The recent trend toward federal deregulation was seen as detrimental to good nursing home care. As a consequence of this movement, the incentive has been removed for improving the health of nursing home patients. It was suggested that nursing homes should be required to operate as nonprofit institutions in a manner analogous to that currently required of hospitals.

Without question, the most effective means of protecting the interests of the young and the elderly with respect to adequate nutritional support is by influencing political decision making. The American Association of Retired People (AARP) is a very powerful lobby on age-related issues such as Medicare and Social Security. On issues not related to age per se the AARP has divided opinions, as is the case in the general population. The Children's Defense Fund (CDF) is a well-articulated, strong lobby on issues related directly to the welfare of children. Of late, the AARP and the CDF have combined their efforts on some age-related issues. There are other concerns, such as agricultural production and food import/export, on which it would be well for the AARP and the CDF to join with other groups to increase the effectiveness of their lobbying efforts. Such associations have worked well for other groups on a temporary basis when issues were clearly defined.

Finally, the claim was discussed as raised by health food groups that agricultural soils are becoming depleted of nutrients at an increasing rate and that chemical fertilizers produce foods that are nutritionally inferior to foods raised on soils to which natural fertilizers have been applied. Without question, nutrients removed by crops must be returned to the soil; however, no scientific basis exists to demonstrate nutrient inferiority of crops from chemically fertilized soils. Nutrient enrichment of soils has been accomplished by the use of mineral and petroleum-derived fertilizers. Indeed, it was pointed out that without this practice, no significant crop yield could be achieved, and this condition would lead to widespread famine. In view of the high cost and broad dependence of U.S. agriculture on petroleum products, a number of alternative approaches are currently being explored. These include experimentation with substitutes for traditional fertilizers, improvement through genetic engineering of the ability of plants to use applied nutrients more effectively, and greater efficiency in the introduction of nitrogen in the soil by nitrogen-fixing plants such as alfalfa.

Reference

1. Malina, R.M., Savaleta, A.N. Secular trends in the stature and weight of Mexican-American children in Texas between 1930 and 1970. *Am. J. Phys. Anthropol.* 52:453–461, 1970.

Summation

Edwin W. Haller, Ph.D.
Gerald E. Cotton, M.D.

Discussions at this symposium have examined the nutritional needs of the young and the elderly in health and disease. Special attention was devoted to the social responsibilities that must be met in order to ensure that adequate nutrition is provided for young and old. The symposium's participants reached a number of conclusions, which are presented here.

Ample nutrition is particularly important in early life, since effects of childhood malnutrition may become evident as long as sixty years later. Some foods are thought to influence the prevalence of various malignant neoplasms, such as carcinoma of the stomach. Low-cholesterol diets begun at an early age have been suggested to decrease the incidence of hypertension, stroke, and coronary heart disease in later life. Finally, starvation ketosis and the fetal alcohol syndrome are important nutritionally related causes of congenital abnormalities.

With few exceptions, the nutrition of the young in the United States is good. Growth failure is more apt to be due to chronic disease than to nutritional deficiencies. When nutrition is inadequate, insufficient dietary iron is the most common lack. Among subgroups at risk, the pregnant teenager from a low-income family is the most likely victim.

Two major causes of abnormal nutrition in the young were identified: vegetarianism and anorexia nervosa. Vegetarians risk deficiencies of vitamins B_2 and B_{12}, calcium, iron, and zinc. If adequate supplies of these substances are provided, the vegetarian diet may be the basis for a long, healthy life. The incidence of anorexia nervosa is apparently increasing, and health professionals should become thoroughly familiar with its diagnostic features, especially compulsion for overactivity. The classic form of the disease has the best prognosis. Poor prognosis is associated with low socioeconomic class, late onset of the disease, excessive weight loss, premorbid obesity, prolonged duration of the illness, behavior disorders of childhood, parental depression, continued poor perception of body dimensions, persistent overeating and vomiting, and lack of motivation. Particularly poor results have been reported for treatment of male patients with anorexia nervosa.

The elderly, too, are at risk of malnutrition for many reasons, not the least of which is sensory deprivation. Vision, hearing, taste, and smell all decrease with age. Thus, it becomes progressively more difficult to distinguish good from rancid food, and excessive salt may not be detected. Loss of teeth may lead to poor digestion. More frequent illness with resultant recurring negative nitrogen balance, greater use of medication, needed or unneeded dietary restrictions, and alcohol all have an increasingly important influence on nutritional status with advancing age. Physical limitations, financial need (real or imagined), and level of support from family, friends, and society also play a part.

Despite these factors, the elderly in the United States generally enjoy very good nutrition, as shown by the HANES 1 and 2 studies. In certain subgroups of the total population, however, this conclusion may not be true. For example, dietary risk factors exist for chronic vascular disease, but identification of specific relationships has not been solidly established.

Food fads represent a special risk for both the young and the elderly. The practice of ingesting megadoses of vitamins is a special concern. Vitamin A in minimum daily required amounts may protect against epithelial tumors, but excessive doses may be very toxic. The symptoms produced by vitamin A toxicity are very similar to those of metastatic cancer, which may, therefore, result in confusion in the diagnosis of a condition that the vitamin putatively prevents. Other fads are reflected in a variety of health food quackery. Young people appear particularly prey to false claims, since their lack of training and experience has made it increasingly difficult for them to distinguish fact from fiction. In addition to the fraudulent claims made for starch blockers, procedures such as hair analysis (which has been determined to be scientifically totally worthless) have become popular guides to nutritional, vitamin, and food supplementation. Cultists and perpetrators of misinformation can be recognized by their claims to information that is unorthodox and unscientific, and by claims to "sole insight" or by statements such as "I believe in."

The determination of nutritional status is particularly difficult in the elderly patient, since the available techniques of assessment are not very precise. The existing height/weight tables are especially unreliable for this segment of the population. Serum albumin, total leukocyte counts, triceps skinfold thickness, arm muscle circumference, and urinary nitrogen and creatinine excretions all provide additional, albeit limited, information. However, the imprecise nature of these measures should not preclude their use. Proper interpretation of these measures is aided by taking into account the patient's age, gender, race, and physical activity. Coupled with skillful clinical evaluation, this approach should result in an accurate assessment of nutritional status in most cases.

The nutritional importance of calcium metabolism was emphasized on several occasions. The functions of vitamin D are now understood in considerable detail. Patients with hypoparathyroidism, renal osteodystrophy, and osteomalacia associated with total parenteral nutrition benefit considerably from treatment with vitamin D hormone (1,25-dihydroxyvitamin D_3). It is also known that vitamin D hormone levels in the blood of osteoporotic women are low, and therapeutic use of vitamin D hormone results in positive calcium balance and an increase in trabecular bone volume. Precise use of vitamin D hormone in this condition, however, remains to be defined.

The identification of classes of patients who are most prone to develop malnutrition during a stay in a hospital has recently been attempted. Children, patients with chronic respiratory disease, those with malignant neoplasms, and alcohol abusers are among those most at risk. Public awareness, establishment of clinical nutrition research units, and education of physicians and other health professionals at undergraduate and graduate levels have led to considerable improvement in nutrition for the hospitalized patient.

The relationship of diet to cancer has proved to be a difficult area to study. The etiologic role of tobacco use in malignant disease has been well established, as has the synergistic effect of alcohol ingestion by tobacco smokers in the etiology of oral and esophageal cancer. Many other factors have been studied, including total dietary fat, cholesterol, meats, and fiber. Their relationship to malignant disease remains unestablished and requires further study. Although results are preliminary, vitamin A ingestion in nontoxic amounts convincingly decreases the incidence of epithelial tumors, especially squamous cell tumors of the respiratory tract. There is some evidence that vitamin A may inhibit further development of such neoplasms even after initiation of tumor growth. Green and yellow vegetables containing vitamin A may also reduce the incidence of stomach cancer.

Obesity remains a problem in our society, but it is probably not a health risk factor per se. Its main contribution to shortening longevity is in its provocation of hypertension, diabetes, and hyperlipidemia. In the absence of these factors, the life span is not shortened by obesity. Proper nutrition during pregnancy and attention to eating habits during early life are important factors in the prevention of obesity in childhood. A current fad treatment of obesity, the use of "starch blockers," has proved to be totally ineffective and fraudulent.

Protein-calorie malnutrition is recognized as a widespread condition among children in developing countries. It is less well known that this condition occurs in up to 15 percent of acute care patients in hospitals in the United States, and a similar problem may also exist in the elderly population. However, distribution of and access to food seem to be the major difficulties in this group, rather than a deficiency in the total amount available.

The foregoing comments demonstrate the need for a strong educational component in nutrition programs. Development of such programs should have a national scope, and older people should be involved in the planning process. This would ensure accommodation of certain special needs of the elderly.

The discussions in this symposium have demonstrated clearly that nutrition and health are inexorably intertwined. Ample nutrition usually assures normal growth, development, and good health throughout life. Although the American diet generally satisfies nutritional needs, examination of certain aspects of dietary requirements and consideration of the impact of public policy on the individual have led to heightened awareness of the importance of nutritional care of the most vulnerable segments of our population, the young and the elderly. It has become clear that not only nutritionists but also politicians, economists, planners, and educators are the guardians of the nutrition and health of the young and the elderly.

Index